C000205375

The Weight of
Compassion
& other essays

In gratitude to the discipline of medicine for endowing me with the ability to reason on the basis of scientific evidence, and to the humanities for tempering any intuitive deductions with the sensibilities of compassion and feeling for the human condition.

The Weight of
Compassion
& other essays

EOIN O'BRIEN

The Lilliput Press
Dublin

First published 2012 by
THE LILLIPUT PRESS LTD
62–63 Sitric Road, Arbour Hill,
Dublin 7, Ireland

A CIP record for this title is available from
The British Library.

1 3 5 7 9 10 8 6 4 2

ISBN 978 1 84351 388 9

Typeset by Marsha Swan in 10.5 on 14.5 pt Caslon
Printed in England by MPG Books Ltd, Cornwall

Contents

PART TWO: *The Corruption of Privilege*

Acknowledgments

THE WEIGHT OF COMPASSION would never have come into being were it not for Gerald Dawe, who in his gentle but persuasive way suggested some years ago that I should bring a selection of my non-scientific writings together for publication. Gerald being Gerald did not let the matter rest there; once I had undertaken to draw essays from times past into what I hoped would be a coherent form he was a constant editorial presence. The collection owes much to his guidance and advice and I only hope his belief in the work is justified by their content. The collection owes much to Edith Fournier, who, not for the first time, gave me helpful advice on structure and content as well as applying an eagle-like editorial eye to the text. I am grateful to her also for the translation of the poem 'Mort de A.D.' by Samuel Beckett.

Kieran Taaffe and the late Daniel McGing were receptive to my request for assistance in bringing the past to light through the use of illustrative historical material, highlighting the role in particular of The Charitable Infirmary in the illustrious Dublin School; and I am grateful to The Charitable Infirmary Charitable Trust for its support.

These essays in *The Weight of Compassion* are drawn from many publications dating back to the nineteen-seventies and I am grateful to the various authors and publishers who gave me copyright for text and illustrative material. I am especially grateful to David Davison whose photography has been so important to many of my writings.

To Michael Colgan, my sincere thanks for agreeing to launch *The Weight of Compassion* on the trust of friendship, ahead of his having read the book.

The staff of Lilliput Press – in particular Antony Farrell, Fiona Dunne and Kitty Lyddon – have been most patient and tolerant in seeing the collection into print, and Jonathan Williams has been a kindly Welsh source of encouragement. I am grateful to my daughter Aphria for compiling the index at short notice.

Finally, to Tona, my thanks for her advice, patience and tolerance.

Foreword

IT CAN HARDLY BE a coincidence that when he looks out one of his front windows Eoin O'Brien looks across Dublin Bay – at the seascape hundreds of thousands viewed leaving from and arriving in to the Irish capital; a wonderful vista which carries the private histories of so many. For the sense of historical movement and flux that underpins these fascinating essays is itself rooted in a deeply felt ethical understanding of individual experience. History may well be tidal but the human story in Eoin O'Brien's writing and practice as a doctor is highly tuned to the personal.

The men and women – doctors, writers, artists, actors and scientists – who inhabit these pages are not cut-out 'representative' figures who stand in for large scale ideas on politics or artistic 'movements'. *The Weight of Compassion* is about individual lives. Indeed the bounty of these essays and the intellectual narrative that underlines them is the essential value of individuality at a time when bureaucratic mission statements and administrative 'targets' occlude the much more important human contact between doctor and patient, writer and reader, artist and audience, teacher and student. While the politics of the medical profession are robustly challenged with a series of forthright analyses in 'The Corruption of Privilege' – a phrase that will be long remembered from this book – the critical balance is always placed upon the individual conscience and the individual imagination.

To survive and flourish in spite of difficulties, including illness, political chicanery, folly, and stern tests of one kind or another – such as Samuel Beckett's experiences working for the Irish Red Cross at the end of WW2 or Nevill Johnson's restless artistic journeys throughout England and Ireland in the forties, fifties and beyond – is the moral focus of *The Weight of Compassion*. The book is also a powerful witness to great literary and scientific innovators including Anton Chekhov, Samuel Beckett, Denis Johnston, and Nicolai Korotkoff.

As a collection, *The Weight of Compassion* reveals the work of a widely read and astute scholar whose professional life as a doctor and specialist has been dedicated to the alleviation of pain and suffering and who, as an academic, has spent decades exploring the circuitry of the heart. 'No symbols where none intended.' Precious wonder that Samuel Beckett, along with Chekhov, should prove to be the book's pre-eminent influence, for in many ways Eoin O'Brien, who did so much in his ground-breaking study, *The Beckett Country*, introduces the general reader to their unique company as an equal.

The torment that afflicted so many during the twentieth century – from the persecution of the Jewish minority of Europe to the abominable legacy of land-mines in our own day, to the current plight of medical doctors in Bahrain, to the bureaucratic and social struggle for a 'fit-for-purpose' medical system in Ireland, is viewed with hope, commitment and, critically, an energetic enthusiasm; its democratic vision of what makes a decent egalitarian society possible is inspiring.

Eoin O'Brien expresses his wish in these pages that the essays, 'written at different stages of [his] career', reflect 'a progression rather than a retrospection'. He need have no worries on that score. *The Weight of Compassion* is a spirited, playful, humorous, forthright and impassioned self-portrait of a great Irish man of letters. What makes a doctor *good*, an artist or writer *significant*, a mentor *trustworthy*, authority *just*, an experiment a *breakthrough*, are questions at the formidable core of this timely, necessary and provocative book.

Professor Gerald Dawe
School of English, Trinity College Dublin

Introduction: Influence of the Arts on a Doctor's Life and Work

I WAS PERSUADED by Gerald Dawe to bring together the essays of a non-scientific nature I had written over many years. He sensed, correctly I hope, that there was ample diversity in what had intrigued me outside of scientific medicine to be of wider interest, but I approached the task with some trepidation. I had, it is true, been attracted to write on art and history and on issues related to the generality of medicine rather than its science, which has been, of course, my main preoccupation, but these essays scattered over many years and numerous journals and periodicals had to be collected and then made acceptable for contemporary printing.

The task of assembling the essays into an order that would give the whole a coherence that was not chaotic was more daunting. After all these essays had been written according to the demands of editors and the topicality of the subject to its time; how then could they be given a semblance that might bring to the whole an order that was not contrived? In gathering the essays I had to ask myself on more than one occasion if my interests in the humanities and friendship with artistic talents had influenced me for the better as a doctor, or had I been distracted from what I had been trained to do, namely caring for sick people? This leads inevitably to the question as to what are the essential ingredients that constitute a good doctor? And the answer lies of course in the eye of the beholder insofar as any definition will be influenced by the vantage point from which the view of 'goodness' in a doctor is perceived.

The academicians, whose business it is to train doctors and who are given as many as six years to do their job, will define the 'best doctor' as the one who achieves first class honours and heads the class. To these pundits the qualities of compassion and feeling for fellow man in the doldrums is, as often as not, a far remove in their exegesis of what constitutes a 'good doctor'.

To the patient, however, the academic achievement of the newly qualified doctor will pale to insignificance in the shadow of unkindness or a lack of empathy with the human condition of pain, suffering or hopelessness. And yet this view taken to extremes can be misleading. A dullard full of human kindness yet oblivious to the scientific advances in medicine can be the antithesis of the good doctor for an ill patient. So in pursuing this theme – no extremes where moderation is likely to be the essence of reality!

Then there is the administrative or health-care provider's interpretation of the 'good doctor', and this will focus on getting the job done at the least cost to society; there will be little or no room for the caring spirit or academic excellence, though our teaching hospitals now belatedly pay lip service to the importance of research and scientific advancement. In truth, however, these administrative stewards are driven more often by fiscal rather than altruistic motives. When I embarked on a research path back in the 1970s I moved around the hospital quietly lest I draw the attention of the authorities to the nefarious practices in which I was engaged. I also tended to be discreet about circulating my research publications lest I be called to account for the time or hospital resources dissipated in such endeavours. Now it is common practice for hospitals and universities to levy 'overhead' charges on research projects.

I recall one professor of surgery admonishing me for devoting time to 'high falutin' research pointing out that my job was to look after sick people, and that the hospital needed 'belt and braces men' (the term still irritates me but conveys tersely a philistinic outlook) who would concentrate on what they were being paid to do – and this from a professor!

To the university leaders of academe a 'good doctor' will be assessed on his productive output measured by the only scientific standard that permits the use of the term 'productive', namely publications in peer-reviewed international journals and the impact they are judged to have on science. This assumes, of course, that the university administration understand the complex intricacies of clinical and scientific research, which, alas, is not always so.

What then do organizations dealing in humanitarian affairs have to say about the 'good doctor'? These bodies are plentiful, ranging from small non-governmental organizations to massive bodies, such as the World Health Organization, but all have a common remit, namely the improvement of health in underprivileged countries torn by strife or decimated by poverty. And here we see another quality being asked of the 'good doctor'; he or she should be concerned enough to give of their time and expertise to help the disadvantaged societies of the world rather than being driven solely by career ambition or being obsessed with self-aggrandizement. Notably these sentiments are not peculiar to doctors emanating from affluent societies but also apply to those graduating from the medical schools of low-resource countries who may be seduced by the rewards to be gained in more affluent societies. The dilemma facing an altruistically minded young doctor is that our universities effectively penalize those who are prepared to jump off the academic treadmill to devote time to humanitarian activity.

What does an interest in the humanities do to our definition of the 'good doctor'? I was humbled once by a woman I much admired, Joan O'Sullivan, the matron of the City of Dublin Skin and Cancer Hospital, where I was visiting physician. On seeing an essay I had just published on some aspect of literature now forgotten she said, 'You should be concentrating on medicine and not allow distractions such as this to deter you.' At face value this viewpoint is perfectly plausible, and indeed literary interests did deflect me from my patients at times but no more so, I suspect, than the golf course, should I have chosen to chase a little white ball across green pastures. However, my feeble refutation of her admonishment ignored what perhaps I did not see at the time, namely that literature and the humanities in general can bring a new understanding, a heightened sensitivity, to the harsh realities of being a doctor.

The bodies responsible for governance of the medical profession have, of course, rigid stipulations as to what constitutes a 'bad doctor' and they have constructed rules to ensure that society is protected from deviant behaviour by doctors. These bodies are largely self-governing but increasingly the departments of government responsible for health care are exerting more influence in medical governance if for no other reason than they are paying both the salaries and the malpractice insurance for its employees. So in the end the legal system of society itself decides if a doctor is 'bad'. However, this is the very antithesis of the 'good doctor' and the crux of the problem is how many 'poor doctors' lurk between the 'good' and the 'bad'. It is fair to say that society is not (or certainly perceives that it is not) well served by a self-regulating body, the members of which will not expose colleagues whose performance is below that which society rightly expects and deserves.

Finally there is yet another, often forgotten, view of what constitutes being a 'good doctor' and that is the doctor being true to himself, having the capability to delve into one's self, to deny the apathy of routine from smothering the qualities inherent in simply being 'good'. I am at the close of a career that has spanned half a century and all I know is that I have been a 'good doctor' too little of the time; but I can in honesty say that I have tried to keep an open mind on the subject and to search for influences that might help to make me a 'better doctor', and these have often been at some remove from medicine. And who should have the last word in judgment of my 'goodness' or 'badness' as a doctor? I think it must be my patients – how many thousands I know not – and neither they nor I can be fully aware of the influences that have made me what I am, but to seek and search for these is the essence of this book.

The essays that make up *The Weight of Compassion* were written at different stages of my career and reflect, I hope, a progression rather than a retrospection, which would be all I could attempt if I now wished to write a mere reminiscence on my career in medicine. They are statements of the influences that seemed important to me at perhpas a particular time and as such provide an insight into aspects of development that may in some measure allow future doctors and their mentors to come closer to defining and producing a 'good doctor'.

The essays in *The Weight of Compassion* are confined to those I wrote on non-medical or non-scientific subjects. It would be remiss of me, nonetheless, not to make brief mention of my life-long association with scientific research and, more importantly, to acknowledge my many friends and colleagues who allowed me to participate in clinical research without knowing of my 'secret life', or as Chekov would have it, 'my mistress'.

The advancements in the management of high blood pressure (now recognized as the leading cause of mortality across the world) are mirrored, I believe, in the history of the Blood Pressure Unit that was founded in The Charitable Infirmary in 1978. This unit, the first of its kind in Ireland, was dedicated in name and purpose to bringing the most efficient and up-to-date management of this serious illness to the Irish people, while also being determined to bring an Irish influence to international hypertension research. The latter endeavour was based on the belief that successful research in medical science could only be achieved through collaborative research – there was no longer a place for the scientist or institution to be an island unto themselves. The Blood Pressure Unit at The Charitable Infirmary, later the ADAPT Centre at Beaumont Hospital, published close on a thousand papers in the scientific literature, and presentations were made at international meetings in many countries in all continents of the world.

The Weight of Compassion has 'matured' through a number of drafts, with as nearly as many essays being discarded as have finally been included; it has been distilled from a four-part treatise to a more cohesive, thematic, and hopefully more readable, compilation that pays homage in the first part to those personalities in art and medicine whose contributions to the humanities compelled me to write about and research their endeavours in more detail, with the second part consisting of essays that reflect my involvement in humanitarian activities and how that influence was to alter my perception of medical decorum and behaviour, which inevitably lead me into conflict with what might be euphemistically called the medical establishment.

The essays in the first part were influenced by personalities I knew and admired. I have always respected talent, be it in music, painting, literature or science. As a doctor I have had to care for many gifted people and this has brought me to appreciate how their sensitivities and needs are unique, often very demanding, but always, in my opinion deserving attention, if for no other reason than that the demands of being endowed with a particular talent brings with it an imperative to serve the genius; the struggle between obligation and the eccentricities that so often comprise the persona of the intellectual can, whether successful or not, result in a tortuous and painful odyssey, which may see the talent dissipated more often than it thrives. A doctor can accompany an artist on this odyssey, and if he is appreciative of the pain of the struggle for achievement and expression, he can provide solace with advice and medical support.

In revisiting these essays many years after their execution I can be critical, of course, of style and the quality of prose, but not of the content or time spent in attempting to capture something of genius and personality. Each friendship left me changed in many ways, that are not always easy, nor indeed possible, to determine.

PART ONE

The Weight of Compassion

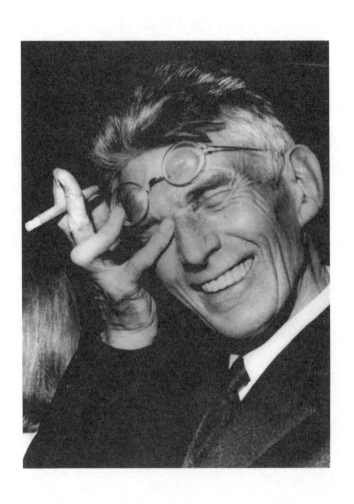

Samuel Beckett

I FIRST MET Samuel Beckett in October 1977. I had sensed in Beckett's writing an Irishness that was most manifest in humour and dialogue, personality and place. However, this essential characteristic was not being acknowledged in the rapidly growing secondary literature on his work. I began researching place and terrain and the inferences of subtle and often occult humour in the Beckett *œuvre*, appropriately on my bicycle, and, what had started as an inkling, soon became a daunting reality.

I discussed this with Con Leventhal, who readily agreed with my thesis and said that I should meet Sam to seek his views. Our first of many meetings took place in the Café de Paris in the PLM Hotel on boulevard Saint Jacques. We began by discussing Alan Thompson, who had been my mentor in medicine and for whom I had cared during his last illness. He had remained, with his brother Geoffrey, a close friend of Sam's throughout his life and he had cared for Beckett's family. Sam was particularly keen to know about his widow Sylvia, with whom I remained in close contact, and his sons Geoffrey, Marcus and Piers. I wondered if we would ever get round to talking about his writing, which I believed (erroneously as I would later learn) should not be an item of discussion unless broached at his behest. Eventually he said, 'Con tells me that you are a cycling authority on the topography of my past!' I then told him I thought the critics had failed to see the relevance of Ireland in his work and that I believed much of the apparently surrealistic in his writing was linked with the reality of existence, and that much of this actuality emanated from his memories of Dublin – or words to that effect; he seemed intrigued by my reasoning. It was I think, a Japanese treatise on the deep surrealism of a passage from *Company* that evoked a warm chuckle in the Café de Paris:

> Nowhere in particular on the way from A to Z ... As if bound for Stepaside. When suddenly you cut through the hedge and vanish hobbling east across the gallops.

To the reader unaware that a place with the remarkable name Stepaside actually existed and, given the context of the piece, a surrealistic interpretation was, of course, quite reasonable, and indeed the very name allowed Beckett to cast a mantle of unreality over the prose.

To my surprise he agreed wholeheartedly with what I was doing and he encouraged me to persist with 'the project', offering to help if assistance was needed: 'Just make me a sign!' We parted on this happy note and my researches now became more detailed, more intense – researches that would lead ultimately to the publication of *The Beckett Country: Samuel Beckett's Ireland* a decade later to celebrate his eightieth birthday. He often became quite engrossed in the memories of times past and he asked me from time to time for details of place names around Foxrock. I recall him having a particular fascination for the name Ballyoghan, which I researched at some length. I did not trouble him for explanations of the obvious in my researches and there were times when I had to leave the obscure anchored in obscurity.

I made many trips to Paris bearing hundreds of photographs so that between us we could select the fraction that was ultimately used in the book. Those days walking through the Luxembourg Gardens with 'Beckett on my back' are full of warm memories – it was a wonderful period in my life. On one poignant visit I produced a photograph of Bill Shannon, the 'consumptive postman' in one of Beckett's most beautiful pieces of prose in *Watt*: 'The crocuses and the larch turning green every year a week before the others ... and the consumptive postman whis-tling The Roses Are Blooming in Picardy ...' This photograph brought tears to his eyes and I realized it was time to bid farewell, pack my bag of photographs and slip away without words, just a hand on his shoulder to show I understood and would return anon.

On another occasion, I laid out David Davison's wonderful photographs of the storm-lashed Dún Laoghaire pier and the anemometer 'flying in the wind' in *Krapp's Last Tape*. Sam confided to me, not quite apologetically but rather in the tone of one who had pulled a fast one and is proud of having done so, that the revelatory moment – that moment when he 'saw the whole thing at last' – had taken place on the much more humble pier at Greystones harbour on a black stormy night when he had been staying in the house his mother had rented in this then seaside resort.

The Beckett Country started life well with a tribute from Samuel Beckett that read: 'My gratitude for this kindly light on other days.' This tribute was extended, not only to me, but also to the loyal team that had made the book a reality against many odds – my wife Tona, Ted and Ursula O'Brien, David Davison, Bobby Ballagh, Kieran Taffee, Pat Lawlor, and the late Harry O'Flanagan.

The popularly held view that Sam did not read anything that was written about him was not quite true as I found out on one occasion to my cost. A photographic exhibition based on *The Beckett Country* was designed to celebrate Sam's eightieth birthday and was first displayed at the University of Reading in May 1986 with readings by the late Dame Peggy Ashcroft and Ronald Pickup.[1] James Knowlson and I published a book to accompany the exhibition, which I sent to Sam. When I visited him a week later in Paris I noticed that he had a grubby brown cloth bag with him and after some pleasantries he withdrew the book – the only content – from the bag and opened it at page 14 saying hesitatingly, 'Eoin, I cannot reconcile this quotation from *Watt* with the original publication and I have even checked back to the manuscript.' I paled as we unravelled a curious happening. The piece of prose in *Watt* that describes Watt's journey on the train from Harcourt Street to Foxrock was read thus to me by Sam:

> The racecourse now appearing, with its beautiful white railing, in the fleeing lights, warned Watt that he was drawing near, and that when the train stopped next, then he must leave it. He could not see the stands, the grand, the members', the people's, so ? when empty with their white and red, for they were too far off.

The question mark, as Sam explained, was a device he rarely used, perhaps only when he was tired, that left the reader to find the most appropriate word – but this was too much for a typesetter in Reading who took it upon him or herself to insert the words 'six chairs' so that the passage now read, 'He could see the stand, the grand, the members', the people's, so six chairs when empty with their white and red, for they were too far off.' My planned route from Paris to Dublin (much against Sam's wishes) was immediately changed to Reading where I sought out this compositing genius in vain but established that the proofs were correct and thence to the printers to pulp the entire run and re-print one thousand corrected copies.

5

Though Beckett, with characteristic humour, proposed his own epitaph, perhaps the most fitting tribute to the genius of his work is, I believe, simply to acknowledge that he reached the zenith of expression, 'the sum of the world's woes in nothingness enclose'. We must not see Beckett's enormous gift to humanity as being confined to his power of expression in prose, poetry and drama; we must look further afield to that largely unexplored realm of this talent – to his influence as a philosopher, and perhaps it is here that he holds hand so easily with a doctor in search of some meaning to the suffering of existence. The essays that follow encapsulate for me much of what is the 'heart and soul' of Beckett's writing. The first is 'The Weight of Compassion',[2] which gives the title to the book; the next two essays, 'The Beckett Country: Samuel Beckett's Ireland'[3] and 'Zone of Stones'[4] examine how Beckett's memories of Ireland, and in particular South Dublin, may have influenced his prose, poetry and drama. The last essay, 'Humanity in Ruins',[5] returns to the theme of compassion and recounts the remarkable story of the Hôpital Irlandais de Saint-Lô where Beckett served as storekeeper and translator along with many volunteers from Ireland in 1946.

The Weight of Compassion, 1990

THERE ARE MANY facets to Samuel Beckett's writing – humour, despair, love, poignancy, suffering – but for me there is one dominant characteristic: *compassion*, compassion for the human condition of existence. What I propose is to illustrate the influence of this pervading quality and in so doing show that this tenderness was present from the moment Beckett first took pen to paper. It is this compassion, tempered, as it so often is, with humour, that makes the suffering Beckett felt for fellow man bearable for the reader. In making this observation we should spare a thought for the pain Beckett had to endure to portray so vividly the state of the world and man's, at times, heroic ability to contend.

Beckett's confinement to Ireland occurred during a period of his life when influences are formative and lasting; a period when the culture, mannerisms and eccentricities of one's society are not only fundamental to the development of personality, but may provide also the raw material of creativity should a sensitive talent be among its youth. To feel compassion, as Beckett did so forcefully, for fellow man is one thing, to express it another. At least two moments on Beckett's path to realization can be highlighted here, each of which illuminate in differing ways the magnitude of the task he was to impose upon himself. The first in terms of chronology (though not publication) is recounted in *Krapp's Last Tape* where the location is readily identifiable in the early draft of the play as the large granite pier at Dún Laoghaire:

> Spiritually a year of profound gloom and indigence until that memorable night in March, at the end of the jetty, in the howling wind, never to be forgotten, when suddenly I saw the whole thing. The vision at last. This I fancy is what I have chiefly to record this evening, against the day when my work will be done and perhaps no place left in my memory, warm or cold, for the miracle that … (*hesitates*) … for the fire that set it alight. What I suddenly saw then was this, that the belief I had been going on all my life, namely – (*Krapp curses, switches off, winds tape forward, switches on again*) – great granite rocks the foam flying up in the light of the lighthouse and the wind-gauge spinning like a propeller, clear to me at last that the dark I have always struggled to keep under is in reality my most – (*Krapp curses louder, switches off, winds tape forward, switches on again*) – unshatterable association until my dissolution of storm and night with the light of the understanding and the fire …

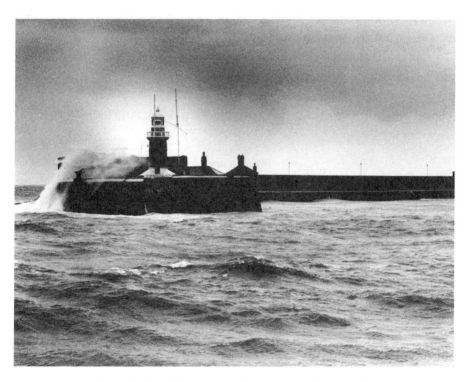

Dún Laoghaire lighthouse and anemometer (D. Davison).

The second moment of realization arose out of his wartime experiences in France, among which the period spent in Saint-Lô with the Irish Red Cross Hospital was to leave lasting impressions. Beckett served as storekeeper and translator to the complex of huts established by the Irish Red Cross in this Normandy town, which had been annihilated by an Allied bomb blitz in June 1944. Here Beckett, and his Irish medical compatriots, saw and shared the suffering of a devastated community. Beckett often discussed Saint-Lô with me, curious as to the fate of those doctors and nurses with whom he had served, and many of whom became colleagues of mine in later years.

From these discussions I came to realize how deeply he had been affected by his experiences there. I never sought, and none can ever know (perhaps not even Sam himself) the abstract influences of Saint-Lô in his writing. There are, however, two works that arise directly from Saint-Lô – a poem simply entitled 'Saint-Lô' and a prose piece, which was written for Radió Éireann; whether or not it was ever broadcast is not known. The pervading sense of compassion, not only for the impoverished people of Saint-Lô, but also for his compatriots, for their naiveté, their difficulty in grappling with the immense tragedy of war, is evident from this emotive report.

That moment on the pier may have fired Beckett's literary vision, but the fulfilment of its arduous demands had to be defined, clarified, and then gathered into a true *vade mecum*, to drive him unerringly and relentlessly towards the achievement of what then seemed the unattainable. This, Beckett did in the remarkable 'Tailpiece' to *Watt*:

> who may tell the tale
> of the old man?
> weigh absence in a scale?
> mete want with a span?
> the sum assess
> of the world's woes?
> nothingness
> in words enclose?

That Beckett should have postulated so demanding an avocatory vision was astounding; that he had the courage and discipline to fulfil it in every detail is testimony to the magnificence of his achievement. Once the course was charted, the process of drawing on the past began, and what treasures Beckett's prodigious memory was to provide for his writing! Back, back to childhood (and at times beyond), to the mosaic of compassion woven from the developmental threads of the people who occupied a growing child's world, tiny when viewed from afar, a metropolis when seen from within.

The coincidence of Beckett's arrival on Good Friday, 13 April 1906 with the remembrance of an auspicious departure could, if taken at face value, be dismissed lightly, or even misinterpreted as an example of Beckettian humour, but no, its profundity is deliberate and those who ignore, or demean this, fail to appreciate the morality that is central to all Beckett's work. I have written somewhere that Beckett's writing is for me more beautiful, more edifying, than the Bible. This is not to demean one of the greatest works we own, but rather to make the point that time changes our perception of great works and with this our ability to be moved and influenced by them. In likening Beckett's work to the Bible, I do so only to state its profound morality and not to impart an unwelcome religiosity on Beckett – Sam was a non-believer, who saw all too clearly the pain inflicted by the intolerance of religion on mankind – his was a message of tolerance.

> You were born on an Easter Friday after long labour. Yes I remember.
> The sun had not long sunk behind the larches. Yes I remember.
> Or if only, You first saw the light and cried at the close of the day when
> in darkness Christ at the ninth hour cried and died.

Beckett's childhood was a happy one and he cherished its memories, which recur in his work, often with greater force and poignancy in his later writing. Foxrock was then a rural, untroubled hamlet. 'In such surroundings,' he wrote, 'slipped away my last moments of peace and happiness.' The smallest incidents, the most insignificant characters were given heroic proportions:

> The crocuses and the larch turning green every year a week before the others
> and the pastures red with uneaten sheep's placentas and the long summer days
> and the new-mown hay and the wood-pigeon in the morning and the cuckoo
> in the afternoon and the corncrake in the evening and the wasps in the jam
> and the smell of the gorse and the look of the gorse and the apples falling
> and the children walking in the dead leaves and the larch turning brown a
> week before the others and the chestnuts falling and the howling winds and
> the sea breaking over the pier and the first fires and the hooves on the road
> and the consumptive postman whistling The Roses Are Blooming in Picardy
> and the standard oil-lamp and of course the snow and to be sure the sleet and
> bless your heart the slush and every fourth year the February debacle and the
> endless April showers and the crocuses and then the whole bloody business
> starting all over again.

Such, in fact, was the pastoral tranquillity of Foxrock, nestling at the foothills of the Dublin Mountains, that on certain spring evenings it became 'a matter of some difficulty to keep God out of one's meditations'. But this peaceful harmony between land, sky, and youth was shattered betimes by the suffering that lurked at every corner if one chose to see it. One growing boy saw clearly and was moved by the tragic figures around him; he observed them carefully in their decrepitude and later restored their dignity:

> In the ditch on the far side of the road a strange equipage was installed: an old high-wheeled cart, hung with rags. Belacqua looked around for something in the nature of a team, the crazy yoke could scarcely have fallen from the sky, but nothing in the least resembling a draught-beast was to be seen, not even a cow. Squatting under the cart a complete down-and-out was very busy with something or other. The sun beamed down on this as though it were a new-born lamb. Belacqua took in the whole outfit at a glance and felt, the wretched bourgeois, a paroxysm of shame for his capon belly.

The down-and-out in many guises is recognized as central to the Beckettian theme. Tramps and dishevelled figures illustrate theatre programmes, books by, and books about Beckett; yet such images are but a shallow representation, a one-dimensional view, of the whole. Deprived of the words that express Beckett's compassion, such pictures cannot impart the sense of dignity with which Beckett has endowed his tragic creations. A picture, however, tender and evocative, cannot convey the poignancy of Beckett's childhood beggar woman:

> An old beggar woman is fumbling at a big garden gate. Half blind. You know the place well. Stone deaf and not in her right mind the woman of the house is a crony of your mother. She was sure she could fly once in the air. So one day she launched herself from a first floor window. On the way home from kindergarten on your tiny cycle you see the poor old beggar woman trying to get in. You dismount and open the gate for her. She blesses you. What were her words? God reward you little master. Some such words. God save you little master.

When Beckett left the childhood environs of Foxrock to become a student, and later a lecturer, at Trinity College, the characters surrounding him changed but the compassionate eyes continued to observe the tragic vignettes of city life that would later influence much of his writing. During this period Beckett lived in a garret on the upper floor of No. 6 Clare Street, where the family business, Beckett & Medcalf, was situated. From here he was within easy reach of humanity, an abundance of which was to be had in Dublin's many public houses. He chose his observational post carefully:

Here he was known, in the sense that his grotesque exterior had long ceased to alienate the curates and make them giggle, and to the extent that he was served with his drink without having to call for it. This did not always seem a privilege. He was tolerated, what was more, and let alone by the rough but kindly habitués of the house, recruited for the most part from among dockers, railwaymen and vague joxers on the dole. Here also art and love, scrabbling in dispute or staggering home, were barred, or, perhaps better, unknown. The aesthetes and the impotent were far away.

In such pleasant surroundings, the proximity of suffering humanity coping, often majestically, with the cruelty of life, became tolerable and provided, more-over, an almost theatrical illusion temporarily blunting the pain of realization:

Sitting in this crapulent den, drinking his drink, he gradually ceased to see its furnishings with pleasure, the bottles, representing centuries of loving research, the stools, the counter, the powerful screws, the shining phalanx of the pulls of the beer-engines, all cunningly devised and elaborated to further the relations between purveyor and consumer in this domain. The bottles drawn and emptied in a twinkling, the casks responding to the slightest pres-sure on their joysticks, the weary proletarians at rest on arse and elbow, the cash-register that never complains, the graceful curates flying from customer to customer, all this made up a spectacle in which Belacqua was used to take delight and chose to see a pleasant instance of machinery decently subservient to appetite. A great major symphony of supply and demand, effect and cause, fulcrate on the middle C of the counter and waxing, as it proceeded, in the charming harmonies of blasphemy and broken glass and all the aliquots of fatigue and ebriety. So that he would say that the only place where he could come to anchor and be happy was a low public-house and that all the weari-some tactic of gress and dud Beethoven would be done away with if only he could spend his life in such a place.

But such reveries were short, necessarily so in the haunts frequented by Beckett, the student. Both inside and out, the pain of poverty abounded; the beggar woman again, this time selling the impossible, seduces Belacqua with the rhythm of her language:

'Seats in heaven' she said in a white voice 'tuppence apiece, four fer a tanner.'
'No' said Belacqua. It was the first syllable to come to his lips. It had not been his intention to deny her.
'The best of seats' she said 'again I'm sold out. Tuppence apiece the best of seats, four fer a tanner' …
'Have you got them on you?' he mumbled.

'Heaven goes round' she said, whirling her arm, 'and round and round and round and round.'
'Yes' said Belacqua 'round and round.'
'Rowan' she said, dropping the d's and getting more of a spin into the slogan, 'rowan an' rowan an' rowan.'

On 31 March 1926, a house named La Mancha, in County Dublin, was found in flames, and six bodies were removed from the blaze: two brothers, two sisters and their two servants. Only the gardener, Henry McCabe, who raised the alarm, survived. A number of inconsistencies in McCabe's account of the event led to his arrest, trial, and conviction for arson and the murder of six people. In passing the death sentence, the judge urged McCabe to spend his remaining days preparing to meet his Maker. McCabe's fate burned on in Beckett's mind, eventually finding expression – a plea for mercy if not acquittal – in *More Pricks than Kicks*:

> Why not piety and pity both, even down below? Why not mercy and Godliness together? A little mercy in the stress of sacrifice, a little mercy to rejoice against judgement. He thought of Jonah and the gourd and the pity of a jealous God on Nineveh. And poor McCabe, he would get it in the neck at dawn. What was he doing now, how was he feeling? He would relish one more meal, one more night.

On long, straight Pearse Street, which permitted 'a simple cantilena' of the mind, many adventures ordained by the Bovril sign dancing 'through its seven phases' were enacted, few more poignant than that of two beggar girls on an evening of human vicissitude in Dublin:

> It was a most pleasant street, despite its name, to be abroad in, full as it always was with shabby substance and honest-to-God coming and going. All day the roadway was a tumult of buses, red and blue and silver. By one of these a little girl was run down, just as Belacqua drew near to the railway viaduct. She had been to the Hibernian Dairies for milk and bread and then she had plunged out into the roadway, she was in such a childish fever to get back in record time with her treasure to the tenement in Mark Street where she lived. The good milk was all over the road and the loaf, which had sustained no injury, was sitting up against the kerb, for all the world as though a pair of hands had taken it up and set it down there. The queue standing for the Palace Cinema was torn between conflicting desires: to keep their places and to see the excitement. They craned their necks and called out to know the worst, but they stood firm. Only one girl, debauched in appearance and swathed in a black blanket, fell out near the sting of the queue and secured the loaf. With the loaf under her blanket she sidled unchallenged

down Mark Street and turned into Mark Lane. When she got back to the queue her place had been taken of course. But her sally had not cost her more than a couple of yards.

The deranged in society, whether they be poor, deformed, or mentally ill, are special to Beckett. As with the poor, he treats the insane with humour, sympathy and admiration, never with disrespect. In madness, the insane sometimes achieve the perfect escape from a chaotic society; no mean feat in Beckett's view. Moreover, absorbed in their worlds, the mentally disturbed are protected from the contamination of society and retain an integrity not to be found in the sane. Asylums are sanctuaries, where the dualities that compose the Beckettian personality are permitted expression and dialogue free of the interference that would necessarily stifle their existence in so-called normal society. Deranged man, for such are those in mental institutions said to be, is given a dignity generally denied him even by the most sympathetic of observers simply because the condition is not *felt*. Though the House of Saint John of God and Portrane Lunatic Asylum feature in Beckett's early writing, and his compassion for the condition of the inmates is expressed in 'Fingal' and *Malone Dies*, it is in the Magdalen Mental Mercyseat, stinking of 'paraldehyde and truant sphincters', that Beckett creates his 'bower of bliss':

> The pads surpassed by far all he had ever been able to imagine in the way of indoor bowers of bliss. The three dimensions, slightly concave, were so exquisitely proportioned that the absence of the fourth was scarcely felt. The tender luminous oyster-grey of the pneumatic upholstery, cushioning every square inch of ceiling, walls, floor and door, lent colour to the truth, that one was a prisoner of air. The temperature was such that only total nudity could do it justice. No system of ventilation appeared to dispel the illusion of respirable vacuum. The compartment was windowless, like a monad, except for the shuttered judas in the door, at which a sane eye appeared, or was employed to appear, at frequent and regular intervals throughout the twenty-four hours. Within the narrow limits of domestic architecture he had never been able to imagine a more creditable representation of what he kept on calling, indefatigably, the little world.

In the pursuit of the quality of compassion, so closely allied to love, one is drawn to Beckett's relationship with his parents. Take the father first, ostensibly shining through history (in the portrayals of those who knew him not) as a simple man, but in his son's writing he rises to a higher plane, if we choose to see it, a plane on which he provides the support so craved for and so much needed by his son in childhood and adolescence:

Yes, this evening it has to be as in the story my father used to read to me, evening after evening, when I was small, and he had all his health, to calm me, evening after evening, year after year it seems to me this evening, which I don't remember much about, except that it was the adventures of one Joe Breem, or Breen, the son of a lighthouse-keeper, a strong muscular lad of fifteen, those were the words, who swam for miles in the night, a knife between his teeth, after a shark, I forget why, out of sheer heroism. He might have simply told me the story, he knew it by heart, so did I, but that wouldn't have calmed me, he had to read it to me, evening after evening, or pretend to read it to me, turning the pages and explaining the pictures that were of me already, evening after evening the same pictures till I dozed off on his shoulder. If he had skipped a single word I would have hit him, with my little fist, in his big belly bursting out of the old cardigan and unbuttoned trousers that rested him from his office canonicals.

However Beckett's relationship with his mother may be misinterpreted by those who fail to appreciate the mores of the Irish family during the first fifty years of the last century, the fact is that Beckett bore deep love for his mother albeit, perhaps, with less intensity, than for his father. Ireland is a land where the spoken word has many meanings and affection often masquerades under the guise of derision. So, in this regard, a plea for 'no symbols where none intended'. May Beckett's death, in a nursing home overlooking the Grand Canal in Dublin, caused her son intense distress, expressed in one of Beckett's most powerful pieces of writing, one which captures not only the profound sense of loss, and relief that his mother's suffering is over, but also the inevitability of death and the timelessness of age, the inexorable cycle of death and birth and life, the whole business of existence:

> – bench by the weir from where I could see her window. There I sat, in the biting wind, wishing she were gone. (*Pause.*) Hardly a soul, just a few regulars, nursemaids, infants, old men, dogs …
> – the blind went down, one of those dirty brown roller affairs, throwing a ball for a little white dog as chance would have it. I happened to look up and there it was. All over and done with, at last. I sat on for a few moments with the ball in my hand and the dog yelping and pawing at me. (*Pause.*) Moments. Her moments, my moments. (*Pause.*) The dog's moments.

My discipline demands compassion and feeling, or such at least would be the public's perception of the 'medicine man', as Lenny Bernstein affectionately liked to call us doctors. Paradoxically, the practice of medicine makes the exclusion of sentiment a prerequisite for the survival of self, and the process, begun in early studentship, soon becomes so integral a part of the scientific persona that the dissipated gems of idealism, among which, of course, may be found compassion, become unrecognizable. The years of training, so carefully constructed by our institutions, initially blunt and finally pervert the purity of vocation and the sensibility of youth, essences to be found in most medical students but so few doctors. It is chastening, but not necessarily a balm to existence, to have this protective wall around one annihilated. I can do no better, in closing with a great sense of sadness that the Sam I once knew is no more, than quote what I wrote with a much lighter heart for a *festschrift* for his eightieth birthday in 1986:

> The occasion is too great, my ability to express too feeble, other than to gasp in gratitude, to acknowledge the greatness of his sum, to admit that I for one will never be as before. Whether for worse or better I know not. But changed as no other ever could. Possessing now an understanding of and feeling for fellow-man as no other could inculcate in a long apprenticeship designed to do just that. The problem now is feeling too much. Not being able to go on but having to do so, as only Sam knows how. Man unadorned: ugly, decrepit, depraved, laughing, despairing, majestic in his nothingness, not always without hope. A life spent with humanity in the doldrums but only seen from afar. Now terrifyingly close. Can't endure the pain once not felt, necessarily so. What now? Still gratitude for the profundity of realization. Might not have come from any other. Might never have come. What then?

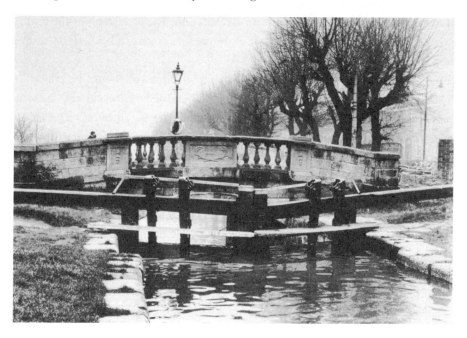

The Hubband Bridge on the Grand Canal (N. Johnson).

The Beckett Country, 1986

THE SEEDS FOR *The Beckett Country; Samuel Beckett's Ireland* were sown, I suspect, when I read *Murphy*, my first taste of the Beckett *œuvre*. After this, I was compelled to read everything Beckett had published. I found myself drawn back irresistibly time and again to one work after another, relishing new sensations at each visit, seeing in the prose or poetry (distinction between the two is not always possible in Beckett's writing), at one time pathos and humour, at another beauty and outrage. Then the works began to blur as the one blended into the other, so that I could no longer, and still cannot (many readings later), always determine the origins of a particular piece of prose. This no longer upsets me, for I now view Beckett's writing as a total composition, each work being a different treatment of sensation, event or emotion, originating often from a single experience.

With this realization, came another. Much of the apparently surrealistic in Beckett's writing is linked, sometimes forcefully, often only tenuously, with the reality of existence, and much of this actuality emanates from Beckett's memories of Dublin, a world he renders almost unrecognizable as he removes reality from his landscape and its people (while also annihilating time) in his creation of the 'unreality of the real'. Compelling though this reality is in Beckett's writing, an awareness of that reality serves only one function, albeit an important one, in that it marks a point of commencement for Beckett's creative art. An obsessional diligence in identifying realities could blight the creative beauty of Beckett's imagination – the 'soul-landscape'.

Samuel Beckett is an Irishman. This simple statement should be taken for what it is, a mere declaration of fact. It should not be seized upon by the patriotic purveyors of national character and genius for public display. Beckett's nationality, taken at face value, is nothing more than an accident, as a consequence of which he was brought up in a small island with a people peculiar to that region. But there is more to it than that. Beckett's confinement to Ireland occurred during a period of his life when influences are formative and lasting; a period when the culture, mannerisms and eccentricities of a particular society are not only fundamental to the development of personality, but may provide also the raw material of creativity should a sensitive talent be among its youth.

It is these influences that are the concern of *The Beckett Country*. I approached my task aware, however, that artistic issues relative to place and person must be interpreted with great care and, never more so, than with Beckett.

Beckett has a justified abhorrence of anyone attributing to minutiae a personal significance that does not, or did not exist, and this has greatly influenced the structure of my book, which concerns itself more with topography than with personality, more with the ambience of a life-style than with those who participated in that life. *The Beckett Country* is not biographical; if it veers towards the genre of biography it is then closer to autobiography, in that it allows the story of Beckett's life to unfold in the only way with which he would be in agreement, that is through his art. Yet, to treat Beckett's writing as a whole as autobiographical would be to reduce its artistic value, and to detract from its beauty.

Proust (a figure whose technique bears a much closer resemblance to Beckett's than that of Joyce) sees art 'put together out of several intercalated episodes in the life of the author', and this is certainly as true for Beckett as it was for Proust. The inspirational influences of time past on the art of Samuel Beckett constitute the dominant theme of *The Beckett Country*. The 'posse of larches' is every bit as potent as the 'madeleine' was to Proust, the granite rocks of Dún Laoghaire pier as revelatory to Beckett's art as the granite kerbstone on the Guermantes pavement was in awakening in Proust the vision that inspired his masterpiece.

I believe that knowledge of the geography and custom of a writer's habitat may enhance appreciation of his art. Indeed Sighle Kennedy goes so far as to suggest that 'entry to certain spirals of his [Beckett's] art will continue to require the possession (in sympathy at least) of a green Eire passport'. I take support for this view also from Martin Esslin, who sees in Beckett's poetry a compression almost to the point of being in code, and this analogy could be extended to much of the later prose:

> A single line may carry multiple meanings, public and private allusions, description and symbol, topographic reference, snatches of overheard conversation, fragments in other languages, Provencal or German, the poet's own asides ... learned literary allusions together with brand names of cigarettes or shop signs in Dublin. Four lines may thus require four pages of elucidation, provided, that is, that the full information were at hand ...

Perhaps *The Beckett Country* will provide some of that necessary information.

Twenty years ago the late Con Leventhal, Beckett's close friend and confidant, identified in Beckett scholarship the neglect of the visual, that aspect of art which Beckett himself prizes so highly: 'In parenthesis and a new paragraph may I ask when are we going to have an illustrator of B's work? Both Blake and Dali have interpreted Dante; it would require a mixture of both their qualities, a power of illumination plus magic.' Con had a painter in mind and one of considerable genius at that; I decided instead to endow the Beckett country with a visual perspective through the art of photography. The portrayal of that land could only be achieved by an artist willing to familiarize himself with the terrain, its people and its fickle sky and light. I was fortunate in obtaining the support of David Davison, who developed an empathy with the mood of the land and the Beckettian character. Together, we walked this land, often returning many times to a particular place to catch the moment when light, sky and object were in harmony with the Beckett spirit, a harmony that was to be further enriched by the delicate manipulation of processing techniques, to create through the art of photography a series of compositions that would be a tribute to the writer who had inspired them.

In spite of a massive secondary literature, it is early days in Beckett scholarship. As is customary, the Irish academic beacon (with a few honourable exceptions), has been directed elsewhere, with the result that the specifically Irish references in Beckett's writing have, for the most part, passed unnoticed. But in the face of such few Irishmen as are aware of Beckett's Irishness, there are those who, whilst in no position to deny him the facts of his birth, nevertheless do not consider him to be truly Irish. The reasons traditionally cited are his Anglo-Irish origins and education, his prolonged absence from the homeland (though allowances seem to have been made for Joyce in this regard), his adoption of a foreign tongue, and the fact that his writings are at variance with the popular pieties of Irish literature.

Beckett's adoption of France as a homeland does not lessen the relevance of Ireland to his writing. He left Ireland for good reasons, having found himself at odds with the canons of propriety. Moreover, the inebriating ambience of Dublin had lain to rest many a budding flower, in 'lakes of boiling small-beer'. Nor should his physical departure from Ireland be equated with a spiritual exodus. He brought with him to France the tools of his trade, the back-drop against which his dramas would be acted out, his models and their dialogue to be spliced on occasion to another language, their aspirations and despairs. He did not as one critic has put it, 'cast off race and genius', and thereby become 'a Frog'. No, as for the protagonist of *The Calmative*, so too for Beckett, 'there was never any city but the one … I only know the city of my childhood, I must have seen the other, but unbelieving'.

Con Leventhal was one who marvelled at academe's inability to appreciate the Irish influence in Beckett's writing. The question as to whether France had the right to claim Beckett as its eleventh Nobel Prize winner in 1969 or whether the country of his birth could claim him as her third (after Yeats and Shaw) drew an interesting comment from Leventhal:

> There is no one here to make the full Irish case. Few to talk of the kinship with Swift though more to tie the Dubliner in a Joycean knot. No one, however, is sufficiently aware of the background to notice the Irishness of the Godot tramps. The highest praise that the dramatist Anouilh can give to *Waiting for Godot* is that in it we have Pascal's *Pensées* played out by the Fratellini

clowns. How could he know or be expected to recognize the Dublin lilt of the dialogue as translated by the author? How few French people were able to realize the added humour and pathos to the French version of *Fin de Partie* when in its English form it was acted by Patrick Magee and Jack MacGowran in the author's own production! The French, ignorant of the exciting possibilities of an *Endgame* played by the right Irish actors, are likewise unfamiliar with the revelatory new touches that these two actors can give to their interpretation of a Beckett text on radio and television.

Any discussion as to whether or not the French or the Irish can lay claim to Samuel Beckett, is of consequence only insofar as it may assist in the interpretation of his work. A squabble over national identity would be most offensive to Beckett, to whom national boundaries, geographical and cultural, have always been tiresome, and at times threatening, encumbrances. Harry Cockerham takes a refreshingly positive approach to Beckett's dual nationality: 'Arguments over whether he is properly a French or an Irish writer are therefore necessarily sterile and it may indeed be that his example and the fact of his existence as a bilingual writer will do much to break down barriers between national cultures and encourage a trend towards comparativism in literary studies.' So while allowing that Beckett is Irish in origins, in manners, and at times thought, we must accept that he belongs to no nation, neither to France nor to Ireland; if any claim has validity, it is that he represents in outlook the true European, but even this tidy categorization is excessively constraining; Beckett is of the world.

Topographic references to Dublin in Beckett's writing are numerous. It is widely accepted that *All That Fall* is set in Foxrock, but what is not so well known is that *Happy Days* may have had its origins in a seaside cove bearing the delightful name of Jack's Hole, that one of the climatic episodes in *Krapp's Last Tape* occurred on Dún Laoghaire pier, and that a case can be made for placing Vladimir and Estragon's vigil for Godot in the Dublin Mountains. *Dream of Fair to Middling Women* and *More Pricks than Kicks* are set squarely in Dublin, whereas *Murphy* is played out in both Dublin and London. Mercier and Camier spend their time between the city of Dublin, its canals and the Dublin Mountains, and there are Dublin locales to be found in *Watt, Malone Dies, The Unnamable, Company, That Time, Eh Joe, Embers*, much of the later prose, and some of Beckett's poetry. Not all see it thus. Vivian Mercier, while freely acknowledging the influence of Dublin in a number of Beckett's novels and plays, asserts that 'Beckett had brought from his carefully insulated suburban community very little that was usable and durable.' Sighle Kennedy, on the other hand, has not only appreciated that Ireland has a relevance to Beckett's writing, she is aware of its significance to his art:

But Beckett's continued and varied use of Irish materials – a usage persisting through more than forty years of his residence abroad – seems to point to some deep involvement of this material with the central working of his genius … The Irishness in Beckett's work seems part of its vital core: that element which he himself sees as constituting in any work of art its 'condensing spiral of need'.

She appreciates, moreover, the dangers of confusing Beckett's national background with his concept of art, or as he once called it 'the autonomy of the imagined'.

An interesting feature in Beckett's writing is the recurrence of theme and scenes with the same people and the same places, most especially in Dublin, being introduced and reintroduced repeatedly. Beckett is not unaware of this as the end of *The Expelled* indicates: 'I don't know why I told this story. I could just as well have told another. Perhaps some other time I'll be able to tell another. Living souls you will see how alike they are.' But no two treatments are the same. The style, mood composition and technique are so varied as to make memorable each in itself. What has inevitably changed, however, is the age of the artist and, with it, his mood, sensibility and most important perhaps, his power of evocation. When Beckett writes from an experience, he often does so from the moment of that experience and the sensations are of that moment be they those of the foetus, of childhood or of aging man. If, for instance, Beckett writes of a small boy, he does so seeing and feeling as did that small boy. When the small boy writes of an old man we should not necessarily permit our imagination to bring before us a picture of senility, but rather that of a man closer to his prime, for such men appear 'old' to small boys. Or when the child speaks of hills of 'extraordinary steepness' we should not be too surprised as adults to find that the reality is an incline of modest proportions. When Beckett writes of the womb experience he is, I believe, writing out of the reality of his experience, which few of us are capable of appreciating because our memories simply do not permit us to do so and we duly designate such writing as surrealistic.

After nearly half a century of exile, Beckett has developed and perfected his talent through selfless dedication to his art, so that the despairing cry in *Watt* now has no meaning for Beckett: 'for all the good that frequent deportations out of Ireland had done him, he might just as well have stayed there'. Beckett left Ireland, but he has revisited Dublin with the same intensity that Proust returned to Combray. Even in his recent writing, he depends upon the sea, the sky, the mountains and the islands that pulsate in 'a mighty systole'. Here, in the Dublin Mountains and on the seashore of Dublin Bay, lies the real Beckett country, the country that was fundamental to the early novels, faded (but never quite disappeared) from the drama and prose of the middle years, until in his seventh decade, 'the old haunts were never more present'. 'I walk those backroads,' he tells us 'with closed eyes,' but it is those roads and mountains that he sees in his mind.

Zone of Stones, 1996

MY EXPLORATION of the Beckett country began a decade ago. There had been a few hints from Beckett scholars, most notably from the late Con Leventhal, Katharine Worth, Sighle Kennedy, and Vivian Mercier, that an unexplored and exciting terrain awaited discovery in Beckett's homeland.

The geographical extent of *The Beckett Country* is readily identified – it is confined almost entirely to the city of Dublin and the surrounding county, most especially Foxrock, and the coast of Dún Laoghaire, Killiney and Sandycove. The heart of *The Beckett Country* lies in the magic landscape of the Dublin Mountains. There are, it is true, references to other parts of Ireland, but for the greater part these serve merely as topographical locations and they are not a creative influence. Easy though it may be to chart the geographic borders of *The Beckett Country*, the same cannot be said of its place in Beckett's writing. When I began my researches I did so in the belief that I would have to concentrate only on the early prose works and poetry. *More Pricks Than Kicks*, *Mercier and Camier*, *Murphy*, *Watt*, and *The Trilogy*, together with the pre-war poetry, seemed to me to contain all the influences of a place and person that was Irish in Beckett's writing. I was greatly mistaken. The influence of Dublin and its people extends throughout Beckett's work, and though the Irish presence faded a little in the middle period of the fifties when the French influence became dominant, it returned with increasing force in the later writings and is at its most powerful and poignant in *Company* written in 1980:

> Nowhere in particular on the way from A to Z. Or say for verisimilitude the Ballyogan Road. That dear old back road. Somewhere on the Ballyogan Road in lieu of nowhere in particular. Where no truck any more. Somewhere on the Ballyogan Road on the way from A to Z. Head sunk totting up the tally on the verge of the ditch. Foothills to left. Croker's Acres ahead. Father's shade to right and a little to the rear. So many times already round the earth. Topcoat once green stiff with age and grime from chin to insteps. Battered once buff block hat and quarter boots still a match. No other garments if any to be seen. Out since break of day and night now falling. Reckoning ended on together from nought anew. As if bound for Stepaside. When suddenly you cut through the hedge and vanish hobbling east across the gallops.

This phenomenon is hardly surprising. Ageing men recall with greater clarity the events of youth rather than those of later years, but it is Beckett's treatment of this biological occurrence that makes his writing in this regard so unique. There is, for those who wish to pursue it, a most profound analysis of the ageing process in Beckett's writing.

It is over fifty years since Beckett's writing was first published, and time has taken a dismal toll on the city he wrote of with such affection. Even the surrounding landscape of mountain and sea has been altered. So-called city planners have seen fit to fill in much of Dublin Bay and if they have their way will continue to destroy this national amenity that has been taken so much for granted by Dubliners. The foothills of the mountains of Dublin have been swallowed up by a rising tide of ugly suburban houses, and even the inhospitable summits beloved by Bill Beckett and his son have been defaced with pylons and cables. Nevertheless much that is beautiful remains in Dublin and it is still possible on a spring evening to experience the tranquillity of the mountain foothills close to Foxrock:

> Leaning now on his stick, between Leopardstown down the hill to the north and the heights of Two Rock and Three Rock to the south, Belacqua regretted the horses of the good old days, for they would have given to the landscape something that the legions of sheep and lambs could not give. These latter were springing into the world every minute, the grass was spangled with scarlet after-births, the larks were singing, the hedges were breaking, the sun was shining, the sky was Mary's cloak, the daisies were there, everything was in order. Only the cuckoo was wanting. It was one of those Spring evenings when it is a matter of some difficulty to keep God out of one's meditations.

Foxrock, Samuel Beckett's birthplace, though more developed than in Beckett's childhood still retains an atmosphere that is rural, elegant and sheltered. Its inhabitants today, as in Bill Beckett's time, are the successful business and professional citizens of Dublin – there is an air of refined affluence about the place:

> Belacqua was heartily glad to get back to his parent's comfortable private residence, Ineffably detached and situated and so on, and his first act, once spent the passion of greeting after so long and bitter a separation, was to plunge his prodigal head into the bush of verbena that clustered about the old porch (wonderful bush it was to be sure, even making every due allowance for the kind southern aspect it enjoyed, it never had been known to miss a summer since first it was reared from a tiny seedling) and longly to swim and swoon on the rich bosom of its fragrance, a fragrance in which the least of his childish joys and sorrows were and would forever be embalmed.

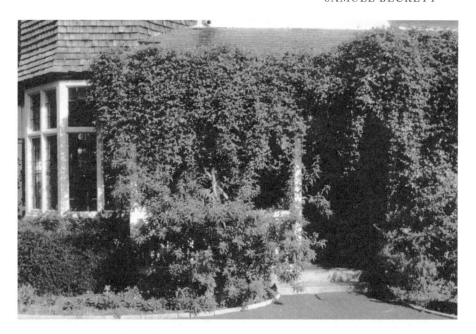

Verbena-covered porch at Cooldrinagh, Foxrock (D. Davison).

In the family home *Cooldrinagh* on Kerrymount Avenue, Beckett grew up in an atmosphere of peace and comfort:

> None but tranquil sounds, the clicking of mallet and ball, a rake on pebbles, a distant lawn-mower, the bell of my beloved church. And birds of course, blackbird and thrush, their song sadly dying, vanquished by the heat, and leaving dawn's high boughs for the bushes' gloom. Contentedly I inhaled the scent of my lemon-verbena. In such surroundings slipped away my last moments of peace and happiness.

Foxrock station, once the focal point of Beckett's childhood village no longer exists: 'The entire scene, the hills, the plain, the racecourse with its miles and miles of white rails and three red stands, the pretty little wayside station …'

Once the pride of the line, as Beckett acknowledges in *All That Fall*, the station is now a derelict ruin on a weed-covered platform astride a track that once carried 'the slow and easy' between Foxrock and Harcourt Street Station:

> Before you slink away. Mr. Barrell, please, a statement of some kind, I insist. Even the slowest train on this brief line is not ten minutes and more behind its scheduled time without good cause, one imagines. (*Pause.*) We all know your station is the best kept of the entire network, but there are times when that is not enough, just not enough. (*Pause.*) Now, Mr. Barrell, leave off chewing your

whiskers, we are waiting to hear from you – we the unfortunate ticket-holders nearest if not dearest.

I walked this derelict line with difficulty from Harcourt Street enjoying the view of the mountains and the gentle intervening plain with Croker's Acres (now the residence of the British ambassador), and Leopardstown Racecourse, happily still with us. Angry residents whose garden boundary was once the railway line now regard the land as theirs and my pastoral thoughts were rudely dispersed on more than one occasion. Deep in what might have been the Molloy country in Shankill, a man wild with anger, cursing loudly and flaying his blackthorn, broke from the woods of his adjoining patch accompanied by his foaming mastiff to dispatch me on my way.

Cooldrinagh, the house in which Beckett was born, still stands, only slightly changed, but the summer-house, in which Beckett's father read his *Punch*, has disappeared: 'There on summer Sundays after his midday meal your father loved to retreat with *Punch* and a cushion. The waist of his trousers unbuttoned he sat on the one ledge turning the pages. You on the other with your feet dangling. When he chuckled you tried to chuckle too. When his chuckle died yours too.'

The larches of Cooldrinagh live on but in depleted numbers, and one still turns green every year a week before the others. The verbena still scents the entrance porch. Connolly's store that features so prominently in *All That Fall* now boasts formica and dralon and a name that is as far from reality as it is from Beckett – The Magic Carpet. Tullow Church and Tully graveyard with its Latin cross exist much as in Beckett's day:

> Some twenty paces from my wicket-gate the lane skirts the graveyard wall. The lane descends, the wall rises, higher and higher. Soon you are faring below the dead. It is there I have my plot in perpetuity. As long as the earth endures that spot is mine, in theory. Sometimes I went and looked at my grave. The stone was up already. It was a simple Latin cross, white. I wanted to have my name put on it, with the here lies and the date of my birth. Then all it would have wanted was the date of my death. They would not let me. Sometimes I smiled, as if I were dead already.

Beckett has even gone so far as to write an epitaph, which if not his own serves at least for the narrator of *First Love*:

> Mine I composed long since and am still pleased with it, tolerably pleased. My other writings are no sooner dry than they revolt me, but my epitaph still meets with my approval. There is little chance unfortunately of its ever being reared above the skull that conceived it, unless the State takes up the matter.

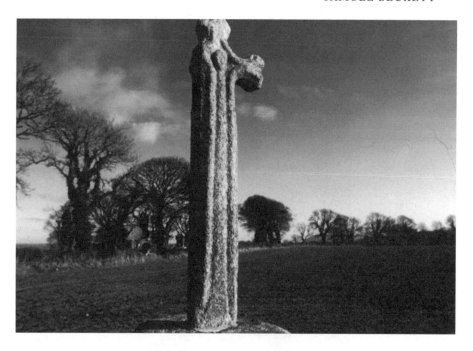

The Latin cross at Tully (D. Davison).

But to be unearthed I must first be found, and I greatly fear those gentlemen will have as much trouble finding me dead as alive. So I hasten to record it here and now, while there is yet time:

> Hereunder lies the above who up below
> So hourly died that he lived on till now

The second and last or rather latter line limps a little perhaps, but that is no great matter, I'll be forgiven more than that when I'm forgotten.

The Foxrock postmen, endearing figures of childhood, are long since dead but not the poignant memories they kindled in a young boy:

But where was the slender one, where was he, that was the question, as thin and fine as the greyhounds he tended, the musical one, a most respectable and industrious young fellow he was, by sheer industry, my dear, plus personal charm, those were the two sides of the ladder on which this man had mounted, had he not raised himself above his station, out of the horrible slum of the cottages, did he not play on the violin, own an evening suit of his own and dance fleetly with the gentry, and, as he lay as a child wide awake long after he should have been fast asleep at the top of the house on a midsummer's night Belacqua would hear him, the light nervous step on the road as he danced home after his rounds the keen loud whistling The Roses Are Blooming in

Picardy. No man had ever whistled like that, and of course women can't. That was the original, the only, the unforgettable banquet of music. There was no music after – only, if one were lucky, the signet of rubies and the pleasant wine. He whistled the Roses Are Blooming and danced home down the road under the moon, in the light of the moon, with perhaps a greyhound or two to set him off, and the dew descending.

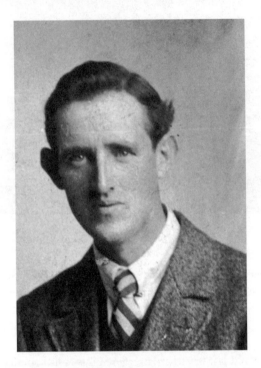

Bill Shannon, the whistling postman (courtesy Mrs Nancy Corcoran).

The identification of place in Beckett's writing is often difficult, an example being a childhood den named Foley's Folly, which is central to the novel *Company*. So dominant is this folly that I knew it had to have firm origins in reality but it proved very difficult to locate. I searched the local historical sources, and consulted with a few reliable historians as to its whereabouts – all without success. On the Ordnance Survey Map of the Dublin Mountains I located a place bearing the name Taylor's Folly. This ruin on the slopes of Two Rock Mountain, once a farmhouse, now houses a herd of pigs, delightful creatures, which consumed my lunch. The view, the overgrown nettles, the solitude (if you ignore the pigs), and the air of tranquillity all seemed to suggest Foley's Folly, but it was well out in the country whereas Beckett states that the den was 'not in the country':

I see a kind of den littered with empty tins. And yet we are not in the country. Perhaps it's just a ruined folly, on the skirts of the town, in a field, for the fields come right up to our walls, and the cows lie down at night in the lee of the ramparts. I have changed refuge so often, in the course of my rout, that now I can't tell between dens and ruins.

When I showed Beckett photographs of Taylor's Folly, he told me, much to my dismay and despite my persuasion concerning the wonderful view, that he had never been there. He remembered however, that the Folly had been originally called Barrington's Tower, but, to use his words, there was no music in that name, so he changed it to Foley's Folly. Barrington's Tower no longer exists as the Folly in the field of Beckett's childhood, but is now part of a fine house, which happily sports a large photographic print of the original tower. Beckett's disregard for the real name of the tower demonstrates that the place of reality in Beckett's work is in kindling the inspirational process, whereas the superficial reality of identification is of no relevance once the deeper reality has served its creative purpose.

We may pause to observe here a striking difference in technique between Joyce and Beckett. Whereas Joyce was fastidious in securing every detail for his literary creation from friends or *Thom's Directory*, Beckett does not generally pay attention to the accuracy or otherwise of his creations, however realistic their source may be. You will say, what about *Murphy* where there are undoubtedly carefully constructed clues to date the happenings in that novel, and there is of course the hilarious request from Paris to Con Leventhal in Dublin to betake himself to the General Post Office in O'Connell Street, to measure the height from the ground to the arse of Cuchulain, whose statue stands in that establishment. This exercise was requested so that Beckett might determine if it would be possible for Neary from Cork to dash out his brains against the hero's buttocks:

> In Dublin a week later, that would be September 19th, Neary minus his whiskers was recognised by a former pupil called Wylie, in the General Post Office, contemplating from behind the statue of Cuchulain. Neary had bared his head, as though the holy ground meant something to him. Suddenly he flung aside his hat, sprang forward, seized the dying hero by the thighs and began to dash his head against his buttocks, such as they are.

But such instances aside, Beckett unlike Joyce is not concerned with embellishing the reality of his creation. For Beckett the reality fires the creative process and having done so has no further purpose; it can, in fact, become an encumbrance in that it restricts the drama to time and place and is better discarded. Beckett is more concerned with tearing away the reality and leaving the creation to stand as it were unsupported in its own beauty; remarkably, in Beckett's hands it does so, whereas the expectation would be for it to disintegrate.

The Beckett boys proved to be accomplished sportsmen at school, and Samuel Beckett was particularly successful at swimming. The sea of Dublin Bay provides the city's inhabitants with a selection of coves and beaches for swimming and Samuel Beckett learned to swim in one of the most beautiful and deepest – the Forty Foot at Sandycove:

> You stand at the tip of the high board. High above the sea. In it your father's upturned face. Upturned to you. You look down to the loved trusted face. He calls to you to jump. He calls, Be a brave boy. The red round face. The thick moustache. The greying hair. The swell sways it under and sways it up again. The far call again. Be a brave boy. Many eyes upon you. From the water and from the bathing place.

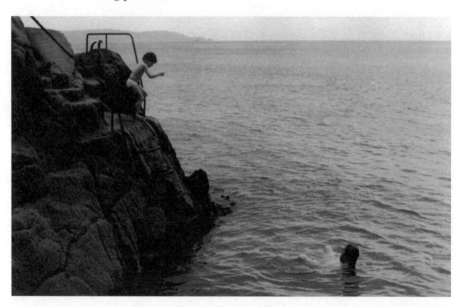

'Be a brave boy.' Father and son at the Forty Foot (D. Davison).

Farther south, the fishing village of Coliemore, and Dalkey Island with its Martello Tower and battery give to the coastline a beauty not devoid of interest:

> The island. A last effort. The islet. The shore facing the open sea is jagged with creeks. One could live there, perhaps happy, if life was a possible thing, but nobody lives there. The deep water comes washing into its heart between high walls of rock. One day nothing will remain of it but two islands, separated by a gulf, narrow at first, then wider and wider as the centuries slip by, two islands.

Important though Foxrock and the close by coast are as influences on Beckett, it is the Dublin Mountains that exert the most lasting and powerful influences. With his father, he tramped these mountain slopes and summits absorbing a terrain that has a unique magic and charm. The mountain peaks with their bog and furze, from which the city of Dublin, Dublin Bay and the Wicklow Mountains are visible in the distance, constitute a landscape that Beckett believes to be unique, a landscape that must endure and influence. He has written of this land: 'The old haunts were never more present. With closed eyes I walk those dear backroads.'

A road still carriageable climbs over the high moorland. It cuts across vast turfbogs, a thousand feet above sea-level, two thousand if you prefer. It leads to nothing any more. A few ruined forts, a few ruined dwellings. The sea is not far, just visible beyond the valleys dipping eastward, pale plinth as pale as the pale wall of sky. Tarns lie hidden in the folds of the moor, invisible from the road, reached by faint paths, under high over-hanging crags. All seems flat, or gently undulating, and there at a stone's throw these high crags, all unsuspected by the wayfarer. Of granite what is more. In the west the chain is at its highest. Its peaks exalt even the most downcast eyes, peaks commanding the vast champaign land, the celebrated pastures, the golden vale. Before the travellers, as far as eye can reach, the road winds on into the south, uphill, but imperceptibly. None ever pass this way but beauty-spot hogs and fanatical trampers. Under its heather mask the quag allures, with an allurement not all mortals can resist. Then it swallows them up or the mist comes down. The city is not far either, from certain points its lights can be seen by night, its light rather, and by day its haze.

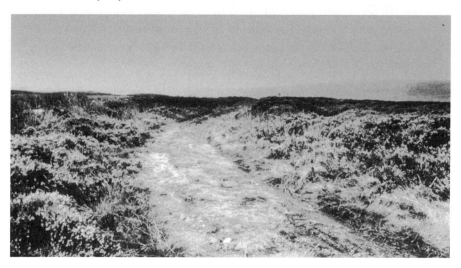

A mountain road on the summit of Glencree (D. Davison).

29

The mountain skies always close to the summit walker vie in their inconstancy of mood with the beauty of the distant views:

> Yes, the great cloud was ravelling, discovering here and there a pale and dying sky, and the sun, already down, was manifest in the livid tongues of fire darting towards the zenith, falling and darting again, ever more pale and languid, and doomed no sooner lit to be extinguished. This phenomenon, if I remember rightly was characteristic of my region.

The water of the bay of Dublin, speckled with islands and ships and fringed by a coastline of rock, rivers and piers, undulates gently its colour in harmony with the inconstant hue and shade of the sky above:

> Even the piers of the harbour can be distinguished, on very clear days, of the two harbours, tiny arms in the glassy sea outflung, known flat, seen raised. And the islands and promontories, one has only to stop and turn at the right place, and of course by night the beacon lights, both flashing and revolving. It is here one would lie down. In a hollow bedded with dry heather, and fall asleep, for the last time, on an afternoon, in the sun, head down among the minute life of stems and bells, and fast fall asleep, fast farewell to charming things. It's a birdless sky, the odd raptor, no song. End of descriptive passage.

The stems and bells of the mountain furze and the ringing of the stone-cutter's hammers in the granite quarries are lasting evocatory memories:

> And on the slopes of the mountain, now rearing its unbroken bulk behind the town, the fires turned from gold to red, from red to gold. I knew what it was, it was the gorse burning. How often I had set a match to it myself, as a child. And hours later, back in my home, before I climbed into bed, I watched from my high window the fires I had lit.

Waiting for Godot is a timeless play. No detail dates the drama or its message to any age. It will adapt to the theatre of the future as readily as it has done to the twentieth-century stage. As it is timeless, so too, it is placeless, demanding little more for its setting than a strange tree, a country road and desolation. Beckett removed most, but not quite all, detail that might permit identification of place in *Godot*. He wished to create, as Con Leventhal so aptly put it, 'a cosmic state, a world condition in which all humanity is involved'. He sought to free us from the restrictions that a specific location would place on interpretation. Beckett did not wish us to see the tramps as 'a pair of Joxers in a limbo of the Dublin Liberties', or a couple of peasants on a country road in Roussillon.

Perhaps then one should desist from even suggesting an influence in Beckett's setting for *Godot*. Might it be better to refrain from touching something so precious for fear of damaging it? And yet …! Walking the summits of the Dublin Mountains in certain weathers the mood of *Godot* is so palpable, that though the urge emphatically to locate the drama there might be resisted, a director in search of inspiration for the ideal setting for *Godot* could not find better than the lonely summit of Glencree, with its occasional threatened tree. Here, Estragon and Vladimir might have settled, as did Mercier and Camier before them. The tree defies accurate description:

> Vladimir: He said by the tree. (*They look at the tree.*)
> Do you see any others?
> Estragon: What is it?
> Vladimir: I don't know. A willow.
> Estragon: Where are the leaves?
> Vladimir: It must be dead.
> Estragon: No more weeping.
> Vladimir: Or perhaps it's not the season.
> Estragon: Looks to be more like a bush.
> Viadimir: A shrub.

I have concerned myself hardly at all in *The Beckett Country* with that favourite of pastimes in the Dublin from which Beckett departed – the hurtful tittle-tattle of gossip masquerading as locutory wit. Beckett's interest in humanity does not concentrate on the individual, nor on nationality, his vision is more universal, he is concerned with the behaviour of mankind, the so-called human condition. Identification of person in Beckett's writing is not generally possible, and if attempted is at best speculative, and not very enlightening. An exception is the important influence of his parents on his writing. Beckett has written, as few others, of the profound influence of his parents on his development. He has done so in a manner that is, to say the least, disarming. He saw his parents as they were with their faults and virtues. He portrayed them as he saw them without permitting either their virtues or faults to colour his literary creation. How critical and intolerant we might expect the young intellectual that was Beckett to have been of a father who had no interest in literature. Content to tramp his beloved mountains, Bill Beckett's love of nature surpassed, in his son's estimation, any so-called cultural deficiencies. This delightful, tolerant, and affectionate man listened to his son, and by listening may have done more to further his development than if he had talked at him incessantly:

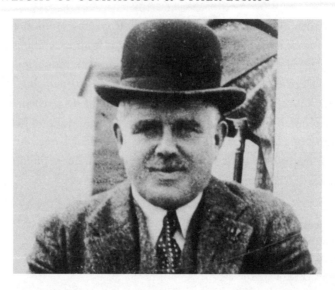

William Frank Beckett at Leopardstown racecourse (courtesy Mrs C. Clarke).

Fortunately my father died when I was a boy, otherwise I might have been a professor, he had set his heart on it. A very fair scholar I was too, no thought, but a great memory. One day I told him about Milton's cosmology, away up in the mountains we were, resting against a huge rock looking out to sea, that impressed him greatly.

The death of Bill Beckett had a profound and lasting effect on his son, who gave expression to his feelings in the poem 'Malacoda'. His father's burial place, Redford Cemetery in Greystones, that 'boneyard by the sea', was a place of frequent pilgrimage for Samuel Beckett:

> I visited, not so long ago, my father's grave, that I do know, and noted the date of his death, of his death alone, for that of his birth had no interest for me, on that particular day. I set out in the morning and was back by night, having lunched lightly in the graveyard. But some days later, wishing to know his age at death, I had to return to the grave, to note the date of his birth.

Humour and affection, qualities, one suspects, that endeared young Sam to his father, disguise the sorrow and sadness that must inevitably have affected Beckett on these visits to Greystones:

> Personally I have no bone to pick with graveyards, I take the air there willingly, perhaps more willingly than elsewhere, when take the air I must. The smell of corpses, distinctly perceptible under those of grass and humus mingled, I do not find unpleasant, a trifle on the sweet side perhaps, a trifle heady, but how

infinitely preferable to what the living emit, their feet, teeth, armpits, arses, sticky foreskins and frustrated ovules. And when my father's remains join in, however modestly, I can almost shed a tear. The living wash in vain, in vain perfume themselves, they stink. Yes, as a place for an outing, when out I must, leave me my graveyards and keep-you-to your public parks and beauty-spots. My sandwich, my banana, taste sweeter when I'm sitting on a tomb, and when the time comes to piss again, as it so often does, I have my pick.

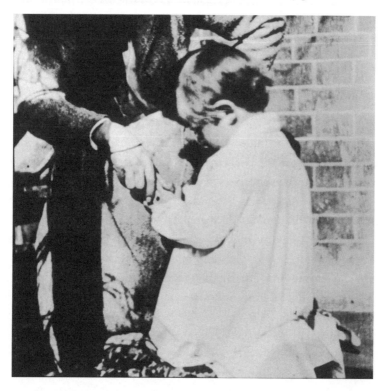

Samuel Beckett at his mother's knee on the porch of Cooldrinagh (courtesy Carlton Lake, Humanities Research Center, The University of Texas, Austin).

Beckett's mother, May Beckett, is often depicted by critics as a soulless, humourless personality typifying the tyrannical and demanding mother so often bestowed on the Irishmen in literature. There may, of course, be some truth in this assessment, but on the other hand, May Beckett did earn her son's lasting affection, even if his patience had been wearing somewhat thin:

next another image yet another so soon again the third perhaps they'll soon cease it's me all of me and any mother's face I see it from below it's like nothing I ever saw we are on a veranda smothered in verbena the scented sun dapples the red titles yes I assure you

the hugh head hatted with birds and flowers bowed down over my curls the eyes burn with severe love I offer her mine pale upcast to the sky whence cometh our help and which I know perhaps even then with time shall pass away

in a word bolt upright on a cushion on my knees whelmed in a nightshirt I pray according to her instructions

that's not all she closes her eyes and drones a snatch of the so-called Apostles' Creed I steal a look at her lips

she stops her eyes burn down on me again I cast up mine in haste and repeat awry

the air thrills with the hum of insects

In interpreting the attitude of the Beckettian character to motherhood, we must bear in mind that in the Beckett country terms such as, 'old bitch' and the like pass for endearment when addressed with affection to the female of the human as well as the canine genus.

Beckett nursed his mother during her last illness in the Merrion Nursing Home close to the Grand Canal. After a night's vigil as he sat exhausted on a bench on the bank of the close by canal and gazed at the window where she 'lay a dying, in the late autumn, after her long viduity', the sign came that she was at peace at last when 'the blind went down, one of those dirty brown roller affairs'. This expression of desire for his mother's death and relief on her passing reflects Beckett's anguish and despair in the face of human suffering, sentiments all the more acute when such suffering is experienced by a dear one, rather than, as some might have it, indifference for or intolerance of his mother.

That May Beckett was a disciplinarian with Victorian principles is beyond doubt, and that young Sam spent many a summer evening supperless in bed, no doubt deservedly so, is clearly recorded, but not in bitterness. Is there not an air of patient tolerance in the delightful garden scene in *Company*?

You are alone in the garden. Your mother is in the kitchen making ready for afternoon tea with Mrs Coote. Making the wafer-thin bread and butter. From behind a bush you watch Mrs Coote arrive. A small thin sour woman. Your mother answers her saying, He is playing in the garden. You climb to near the top of a great fir. You sit a little listening to all the sounds. Then throw yourself off. The great boughs break your fall. The needles. You lie a little with your face to the ground. Then climb the tree again. Your mother answers Mrs Coote again saying, He has been a very naughty boy.

We may even go so far as to say that had the mature Sam Beckett had to deal with recalcitrant progeny, he might have applied far stricter criteria of discipline than May Beckett, if Moran's treatment of his son is anything to go by:

> The dirty little twister was letting the air escape between the valve and the connection which he had purposely not screwed tight. Hold the bicycle, I said, and give me the pump. The tyre was soon hard. I looked at my son. He began to protest. I soon put a stop to that. Five minutes later I felt the tyre. It was as hard as ever. I cursed him.

Whatever the discipline, whatever the exasperation that the young Beckett, in common with all children, may have felt for his parents and perhaps for his mother in particular, the lasting effect was one of a deep affection and a sense of gratitude to which his writing is testimony. There was, I believe, a deeper and more important influence imparted to Samuel Beckett from his parents, and we might for want of a better term, identify this as the Christian ethic. Bill and May Beckett, though devout followers of the Church of Ireland, imparted to their son, not so much a sense of religion, but a truly Christian sense of compassion and charity.

I have concentrated on what I have chosen to call the heart of the Beckett country, the reality that was Beckett's childhood, because the influences from this period are of greatest relevance to his writing. I have left aside consideration of lesser, though by no means unimportant, influences such as school, Trinity College, the people and the institutes of Dublin, because they lack, or only possess in a small degree, that quality that gives to the childhood memories their remarkable strength – namely evocation.

That Dublin is a powerful influence, the point of commencement, in fact, of much of Beckett's writing, is I think quite evident, but that influence in itself would be insufficient to explain the genius of Beckett's talent. After all, many fine Irish writers have this common background but have failed to achieve in their writing that 'something' that elevates Beckett's work to an unusual pinnacle in art. If we wish to examine that indefinable essence more closely rather than merely dismissing it as 'genius', I suggest that it is to France we should look. Not for the French language, important influence though that is, but to Marcel Proust, who permitted Beckett to develop the evocatory sense that allowed him to extract, as it were, the essence from his formative period. The recognizable senses of taste, smell, hearing, sight and touch provided insufficient sensory material for Proust's creative process, which remained impotent until he recognized in himself a latent other sense, a sense that has either atrophied, or more likely has not developed in most of us into a recognizable sense in the terms we employ to define such physiological entities. Beckett appreciated immediately the importance of Proust's discovery of this extra sense that was not dependent on memory alone and which added a new dimension to the creative process. So fascinated was he by this evocatory technique that he listed the fetishes, as he called them, that fired Proust's process of intellectualized animism – the Madeleine steeped in tea, the steeples of Martinville, a musty smell in a public lavatory, three trees, the hedge of hawthorn near Balbec, uneven cobbles in the courtyard of the Guermantes Hotel, and so on.

We can, without difficulty, draw up a list of evocatory stimuli for Beckett as he did for Proust – the larch tree, the smell of the lemon verbena, the granite pier of Dún Laoghaire, the tinkle of the stone-cutter's hammer, and most powerful of all the shaving mirror in New Place. The tenuity of existence and the ephemerality of survival are evoked forcibly by Beckett in the contrasting qualities of a shaving-mirror's material durability and the transience of its reflected imagery:

> I can see me still, with those of now, sealed this long time, staring with those of then, I must have been twelve, because of the glass, a round shaving-glass, double-faced, faithful and magnifying, staring into one of the others, the true ones true then, and seeing me there, imagining I saw me there, lurking behind the bluey veils, staring back sightlessly, at the age of twelve, or at the age of forty, for the mirror remained, my father went but the mirror remained, in which he had so greatly changed, my mother did her hair in it, with twitching hands, In another house, with no view of the sea, with a view of the mountains, if it was my mother, what a refreshing whiff of life on earth.

So though we might say that much of Beckett's writing is autobiographical in that it is dependent on the past – his past – it is elevated above this genre and given an exquisite delicacy through evocation. The achievement of evocation is no easy matter; it does not happen at will; its presence is resented by voluntary memory and the other senses that seek to dispel it; it is, as Beckett called it, 'a discordant and frivolous intruder'. When it obliges, it may do so at most inopportune moments, and intrude though it may; it should be prized for what it is, seized and held for as long as possible to the exclusion of all else. It is the retention of the evocatory state that is so difficult, so draining, but the creative yield from the sensation will, of course, be dependent on the extent of the experience. Evocation permits what science fiction writers dream about, namely transportation in time, regrettably only within one's own time span, but this is, nevertheless, a substantial achievement.

Consideration of this phenomenon may modify our interpretation of Beckett's writing. When he writes of the places, the people and sensations that the evocatory moment permits him, he writes as he feels and sees in the evocation. If it is a boy writing of an old man, the man is 'old' in the eyes of the boy only; that is, he might be no more than thirty or forty or even twenty, but 'old', so old in the eyes of the very youthful observer:

> Where then but there see now another. Bit by bit an old man and child. In the dim void bit by bit an old man and child. Any other would do as ill. Hand in hand with equal plod they go. In the free hands – no. Free empty hands. Backs turned both bowed with equal plod they go. The child hand raised to reach the holding hand. Hold the old holding hand. Hold and be held. Plod on and never recede. Slowly with never a pause plod on and never recede. Backs turned. Both bowed. Joined by held holding hands. Plod on as one. One shade. Another shade.

Hills of 'extraordinary steepness' to the child are to us adults nothing more than mere inclines. Such indeed is the case in the delightful scene with his mother at the first aviation meeting in Ireland in 1910 at Leopardstown Racecourse. Here the hill of extraordinary steepness is Cornelscourt Hill Road a relatively gentle incline:

> But I have heard aeroplanes elsewhere and have even seen them in flight, I saw the very first in flight and then in the end the latest models, oh not the very latest, the very second latest, the very antepenultImate. I was present at one of the first loopings of the loop, so help me God. I was not afraid. It was above a racecourse, my mother held me by the hand. She kept saying, it's a miracle, a miracle. Then I changed my mind. We were not often of the same mind. One day we were walking along the road, up a hill of extraordinary steepness, near home I imagine, my memory is full of steep hills, I get them confused. I said, the sky is further away than you think, is it not, mama? It was without malice, I was simply thinking of all the leagues that separated me from it. She replied, to me her son, it is precisely as far away as it appears to be. She was right. But at the time I was aghast. I can still see the spot, opposite Tyler's gate. A market gardener, he had only one eye and wore sidewhiskers. That's the idea, rattle on. You could see the sea, the islands, the headlands, the isthmuses, the coast stretching away to north and south and the crooked moles of the harbour. We were on our way home from the butcher's.

It is, I think apparent, that much, but by no means all of Beckett's writing has its origins in a real world, and that much of the inspirational energy in his writing emanates from the place of his childhood, which happened to be Dublin. He has rendered this world almost unrecognizable by denuding its landscape and its people (while also annihilating time) in his creation of 'the unreality of the real'. Yet like Krapp, who found inspiration on the East Pier of Dún Laoghaire harbour, so too did Beckett find the inspiration for his writing in this intimate world of childhood. This inspiration was to direct Beckett towards reduction rather than embellishment, towards poverty and decrepitude rather than beauty and possession, towards the land he was soon to depart, the land of his childhood, of sea and mountain, that was to continue pulsating within him in a mighty systole destined ultimately to find expression in the art that has so enriched our existence and our understanding of that existence.

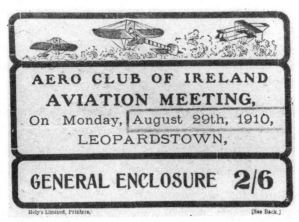

Ticket for aviation meeting at Leopardstown Racecourse, 1910 (courtesy T. Cranitch, Aer Lingus).

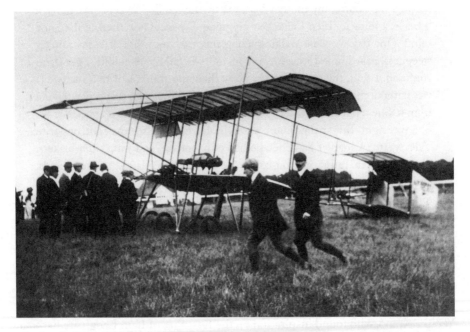

Spectators around a Farman biplane (courtesy T. Cranitch, Aer Lingus).

Humanity in Ruins, 1990

IN 1945 the Irish Red Cross established a hospital in the devastated French town of Saint-Lô. This venture deserves a place in the sun. The experience, which gave to the participants an appreciation of the essence of what is often glibly called compassion, did much more besides; these young nurses and doctors with their support staff felt the warmth of giving and received in return something that rises above the commonly accepted expression of gratitude, the lasting memory of a smile, a flicker of relief on a suffering visage, the last look of despair transformed fleetingly to hope on the fading features of a dying child, all in a French province that had come to know the meaning of suffering. The enrichment and the disillusionment with mankind that was the lot of those who went to Saint-Lô has been expressed, as none other can ever hope to do, by the storekeeper to the expedition – Samuel Beckett.

Alan Thompson and his brother Geoffrey were educated at Portora Royal School in Enniskillen where they formed a close friendship with Sam Beckett. This friendship matured during their undergraduate days at Trinity College, after which their ways parted. Geoffrey went to London to study psychiatry and Alan, after obtaining his postgraduate qualifications, was appointed physician and pathologist to the Richmond Hospital in 1932. Beckett, after graduating from Trinity, went to Paris as *lecteur* to the École Normale Supérieure. Here he met his predecessor, Thomas MacGreevy, who introduced him to James Joyce and an intimate group of writers and intellectuals. After a brief period in Trinity as lecturer in modern languages and five unsettled years travelling in Europe, he exchanged the physical safety of neutral Ireland for the spiritual freedom of wartime France. 'I preferred France in war to Ireland in peace' is an indictment not only of the restrictive intellectual climate of Ireland in the forties; it is a brave denial of neutrality by one who was experiencing first hand the threat of Nazi Germany.

In Paris Beckett joined the Resistance cells, *Gloria* SMH (for His Majesty's Service spelled backwards) and Etoile. In 1942 he escaped from Nazi-occupied Paris and travelled to Roussillon, where he again became involved in the local resistance movement, the *maquis*. (In 1945 he was awarded the *Croix de Guerre* with a gold star by General Charles de Gaulle for his intelligence work in the resistance.) At the end of the war he returned to Dublin and renewed his friendship with Alan Thompson, who was now a senior physician on the Richmond staff. He was also a member of a small team of Irish Red Cross workers engaged in organizing a relief hospital for the bombed town of Saint-Lô in Normandy. Beckett readily accepted an invitation from his friend to join the team as interpreter and storekeeper.

The Irish Red Cross's involvement with Saint-Lô began after the Allied invasion of France in 1945, when the Irish Red Cross offered help to its sister body in France, and representatives from Ireland visited a number of devastated areas. They selected the town of Saint-Lô on the main Cherbourg-Paris line as being in urgent need of assistance. The event was reported in the daily newspapers:

> Irish Red Cross Hospital Experts leave for Paris. Headed by Colonel Thomas J McKinney, Officer in Charge of the Irish Hospital Unit for France, The Irish Red Cross Society's team of expert advisors left Dun Laoghaire by the Mail-boat yesterday morning, on the first stage of its journey to Paris, where the necessary advance arrangements for the unit's reception will be made. The delegation, which with Colonel McKinney consists of Dr Alan Thompson, Mr Michael Scott and Commandant C J Daly, will be met in London and Paris by Eire's representatives and probably will spend a number of weeks in France making a preliminary survey and completing final arrangements.

McKinney wrote of this preliminary visit as follows: 'I had the opportunity to visit France in April 1945, when negotiations were in progress between the French and Irish Red Cross societies to determine what help the Irish could give. I saw Brest, which I reached at night. What feelings I had in this city of silence, gloom and ashes. I saw Saint-Lô, a little later. It well deserved its title, Capital of the Ruins. On my return to Ireland, I had the opportunity of addressing my compatriots over the radio on my impressions of France; I ended the programme with the words "it is imperative that Ireland help France, her neighbour and friend".'

Saint-Lô, a town of some 13,000 people, had served as an important operational centre for the German army. On a June afternoon in 1944, without warning, the Allied forces blitzed the town. So devastating was the attack that hardly a building was left standing, and thousands of citizens were killed. A year later bodies were still being removed from the debris and 3000 people were living among the ruins. The city's only hospital had been destroyed in the blitz. A local correspondent likened Saint-Lô to 'an upturned dustbin' where life began again, almost incredibly, after the Holocaust:

> Life started again in spite of the deadening atmosphere, in spite of the dust, the impassable streets, the darkness, the lack of water and of hygiene, the lack of everything; in spite of the winter with its succession of ills, in spite of the cold which never leaves you, the lack of heating and of shelter in this windy area; in spite of the mud which is everywhere, impregnating those few clothes you have left. Life took up again, but it was exhausting, because the battle against the ruins became also a battle against sickness and death, but to be ill in Saint-Lô was unimaginable, though sadly inevitable for many. There was

no longer a hospital, and the overworked doctors who returned had no place to work and perhaps save lives... In reply to the Health Ministry and the Red Cross, Ireland made the kind gesture of adopting Saint- Lô and brought all that was necessary and more.

The Irish Red Cross offered a hospital unit of 100 beds, and as no building was available for conversion, it was planned to erect wooden huts on the outskirts of the bombed town. The Irish Red Cross undertook to equip, staff and maintain the hospital for as long as would be necessary. The transportation of supplies for such a hospital from Dublin to France was a considerable undertaking, as was the recruitment of medical and nursing staff, the success of which owed much to the hospital's matron, Mary Crowley. In August 1945 an advance party consisting of Colonel Thomas J. McKinney, director of the unit, Dr Alan Thompson, physician, and 'Mr S.B. Beckett, Quartermaster-Interpreter,' left Dublin for Saint-Lô. As well as accepting the post of interpreter, Beckett had also agreed to act as store-keeper to the hospital. Later in the month the *Menapia* set sail for Cherbourg, the nearest port to Saint-Lô, with 174 tons of equipment, six ambulances, a utility wagon, and a lorry aboard. There were special facilities for 'the transport in cold storage of supplies of blood serum and penicillin'. On Monday, 27 August 1945, another contingent consisting of Mr Freddie McKee, assistant surgeon, Dr Arthur Darley, assistant physician, Dr Jim Gaffney, pathologist, Mr Killick, technician, and Mr Dunne, assistant storekeeper, departed from Dún Laoghaire on the SS *Cambria* for London, from where they sailed to Dieppe on TSS *Isle of Guernsey*.

Arthur Warren Darley was born on 23 August 1908. He was educated at St Gerard's School, Dublin, at the Benedictine College, Douai, in England, and by private tuition. His father was a famed musician and Arthur Darley was an accomplished violinist, pianist and guitarist, often accompanying the celebrated Delia Murphy on record. He studied medicine at Trinity College, Dublin, where he qualified in 1931. He spent some time in the Richmond Hospital and two years working among Dublin's poor. In 1936 he worked as 'assistant' at Portrane Asylum with the intention of specializing in nervous diseases. However, in February 1937, 'Dr Arthur Warren Darley shook the dust of Dublin from his feet ... and hied himself off to see the world' as doctor on a Canadian Pacific liner. When the opportunity to provide medical expertise to alleviate suffering in war-torn France arose, Arthur Darley readily accepted.

James Gaffney was born on 1 July 1913, educated at O'Connell Schools, North Richmond Street, and Trinity College, Dublin, where he graduated as a doctor of medicine in 1934, at the age of twenty-one. After a period of training in pathology in Great Britain, he returned to Dublin to an academic appointment with R.A.Q. O'Meara at Trinity College, with an attachment to Sir Patrick Dun's Hospital.

The Irish Red Cross had established headquarters at the *Hotel des Arcades* in Dieppe, where Beckett met the hospital staff arriving from Dublin and drove them through Rouen to Saint-Lô. Dr Gaffney has described his first impressions of war-torn Normandy:

> Coming into Dieppe we got our first view of wholesale destruction … We walked down the gangway and were met by Col. McKinley and Sam Beckett (storekeeper). They had the big Ford VB Utility wagon with them, and after going through Customs we got in. We weren't hungry as we had had an excellent four-course lunch on board and later tea; but nevertheless Sam brought us 3 huge bags of pears, grapes and plums. It was novel being driven on the right-hand side of the road and Sam believes in getting the 150 miles done as quickly as possible. Five miles out of a village like Croagh called St Aubin sur Seine and luckily, just at a garage, a queer noise was heard from the engine and we had to have it looked over by a young mechanic. Sam Beckett is official interpreter as well as storekeeper and although a Dublin man has lived for 10 years in France, so the language is no trouble.

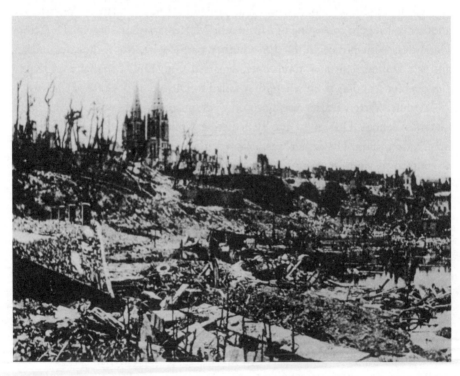

Saint-Lô in ruins (courtesy Miss M. Crowley).

After a night's rest in a nearby village the party travelled onwards by train, leaving Beckett and his assistant Dunne to follow on with the restored wagon. Gaffney has left the following account on his first impression of Saint-Lô:

… It took us about three quarters of an hour to find the hospital. This wasn't surprising, as one street of ruins looks very much like another … Many of the streets can only be traversed on foot by stepping from one pile of bricks to another, or from one rusted girder on to the end of a buried bedstead. Many cellars still lie under the debris and demolition work goes on slowly but surely. Digging the other day, they found the body of one of the local bakers and two of his assistants; and as we arrived we heard the distant explosions of two mines … Of the pre-war population of about 12,000 many cleared out altogether, and they have accounted for about 1,500 bodies, while about 700 remain unaccounted for … The Mental Hospital also is a shell, many of the inmates being killed. In the local jail (which is large) about 29 prisoners were burned to death – locked in, they couldn't get permission in time to release them.

The locals say the Americans dropped HE incendiary and phosphorous bombs on the town; biggest attack was about June 6, 1944, but it was later bombarded by heavy artillery in September. For about six weeks the town kept changing hands between the Germans and the Americans. There are still about 5,000 people in it, but you would wonder where or how they live; mostly in boarded up cellars, on mattresses. Yet, with all their sufferings, they are tackling the problem of reconstruction, cheerfully.

The eight members of the advance team lived together in one of ten huts erected by the French. There was electricity but no running water or sanitation. Beckett, Thompson and Dunne superintended the stacking and sorting of 250 tonnes of supplies, which were brought from Cherbourg by rail and lorry. The store was situated in the lofts over the stables of a stud-farm a half-mile from the hospital. They were assisted by German prisoners of war.

There was little to do when the day's work was complete, other than read, write, and play darts, chess, draughts or bridge. The Colonel advocated a policy of mingling with the local people, and provided expenses for forays into Saint-Lô to concerts, race meetings and the occasional dance. Hot running water was available at an American base thirty miles away where the luxury of an occasional shower was enjoyed. The padre of this camp, Father Bardick, from Connecticut, who appreciated the comforts of life, took the Irish group to 'a magnificent chateau where the Rev. Mother welcomed us and gave a seven-course dinner to the whole eleven of us; got around the piano afterwards and sang for further orders till about one AM. They want us to come again to have a real look around and we promised to do so. Dr Thompson and Beckett said they hadn't thought that convents were such nice places.'

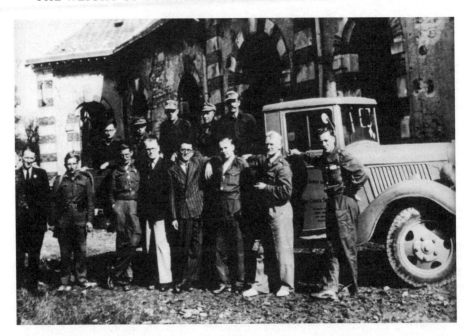

Members of the hospital staff (from left to right): *Dr A.W. Darley, a French military guard, Samuel Beckett, Surgeon F. McKee, Dr J.C. Gaffney, Mr M.B. Killick, Col. T.J. McKinney, Mr T. Dunne. The men in the lorry are German prisoners of war (*The Irish Times *photograph, courtesy Miss J. Gaffney).*

In September 1945 Dr Alan Thompson submitted a confidential report on the difficulties in establishing the hospital:

> It was necessary to find a temporary store in Saint-Lô. We were fortunate in getting a large granary in a Stud Farm near the hospital. When the ship arrived we saw the stores off the ship to railway wagons, and returned to St Lô. After a few days railway wagons commenced to arrived at St Lô. We had to move the stores by lorry 1–1½ miles to our store. Everything had to be taken upstairs. Some packets weighed over 2 cwts. Stores came in for days and days. All are stored safely now. It was a considerable task … The present position is that stores are safely housed under lock and key and well protected from the rain. The Storekeeper (Samuel Beckett) and assistant are making out stock cards for all material … We borrowed beds and camped out in the hut. No running water – no sanitation of any kind.
>
> The water had to be carried in buckets … Sanitation was held up due to lack of pipes and still consists of a hole in the ground with sacking around it. It is impossible, while sanitation is so primitive, to contemplate bringing out any additional staff … The climate is very wet and muddy. Facilities for

amusement are virtually nil … The people seem to be very anxious for us to work there. They are asking all the time when the hospital will be open and taking in patients. The Mayor is very keen on the hospital functioning …

Recreational facilities were improved when the Countess Kerjorley, wife of the president of the French Red Cross, offered a seaside villa to the staff of the Hospital for use in their off-duty time.

Beckett appears to have fulfilled the role of driver, as well as that of store-keeper and interpreter. He drove regularly to Dieppe and Cherbourg to collect supplies and meet personnel, and also to Paris, often accompanied by Gaffney:

Sam Beckett was driving him [Col. McKinney] to Paris on Friday and I had to get my still, so off we went. Sam and I took turns driving a small ambulance and the roads are very good indeed except where there are potholes etc. from tank tracks and small explosions. Driving here is easy and quite safe, I should say, as traffic is practically nil, any cars that are on the road are about 10–12 years old and they do about 25 miles per hour. We kept to about 35–40 m.p.h. and the day was lovely.

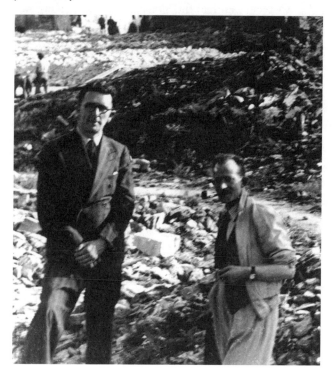

Dr J.C. Gaffney (left) *standing in the ruins of Saint-Lô with Mr M. McNamara, Irish Red Cross Society (courtesy Miss J. Gaffney).*

In Paris, Beckett usually went to his flat, but he did not neglect his Irish friends who were unfamiliar with the sights of the capital, as Jim Gaffney recorded:

> Saturday morning we did some of my business till lunch time and also Sam took me into Notre Dame which was magnificent. Sam has an assistant store-keeper here named Tommy Dunne, a very decent little Dublin chap. Sam is a TCD graduate, interested in writing and in letters generally; he has lived in Paris the last 6 years or 7. He is a most valuable asset to the unit – terribly conscientious about his work and enthusiastic about the future of the hospital, likes a game of bridge and in every way a most likeable chap, aged about 38–40, no religious persuasion; I should say a free thinker – but he pounced on a little rosary beads which was on a stall in Notre Dame to bring back as a little present to Tommy D. It was very thoughtful of him.

The advance party worked tirelessly to prepare the hospital for the reception of patients. Among the first to receive treatment at the new hospital was an eleven-year-old boy who lost three fingers when a hand-grenade with which he was playing detonated. Other advances were also achieved. The first lavatory was installed in October and had the unusual effect of making some of the team homesick. The housekeeper of the Hospital, Madame Pilorgat, brought all visitors to the hospital to view the new apparatus, which she described glowingly as 'magnifique'. By Christmas 1945 the full Irish staff, consisting of ten doctors, each a specialist, thirty-one state-registered nurses, most of whom had specialist training, a pharmacist, pathologist, and administrative staff, had arrived. Between thirty and thirty-five nurses were selected in Dublin: 'Nurses salaries will range from £300 a year (for the matron) to £100 a year (for an ordinary nurse). Staff sisters and theatre sisters will be paid £150 a year. When the nurses have been picked, the Society's team will be almost complete, as already fifteen doctors have been chosen in addition to a number of clerical and technical workers.' By March 1946 eighty in-patients were receiving treatment, and over 120 patients attended the out-patient department.

Finally, all was ready for the inaugural ceremony, which took place on Sunday, 7 April 1946. A Dublin contingent of Mr Maguire (chairman of the Irish Red Cross) and his wife, Dr Shanley, Mrs Frank Fahy, Dr Alan Thompson and Colonel Thomas McKinney arrived the day before the inauguration. The Irish ambassador, Mr Murphy and his wife, the secretary, Mr McDonald, and Miss Maura McEntee reporting for *The Irish Press*, arrived from Paris. On Sunday, the Inauguration Ceremony began at 9.30 AM with mass celebrated by the hospital chaplain, Fr Brendan Hynds, and attended by the officers of the municipality, the delegates from Dublin, the hospital staff and the public. After a banquet luncheon attended by 140 guests, the Gendarmerie with the Band of the French Fleet led a parade to martial music through the ruined streets lined by the enthusiastic citizens of Saint-Lô waving paper Irish tricolours. At the War Memorial in what was once the beautiful Cathedral Square of Saint-Lô, a wreath was solemnly placed on the grave of the Unknown Soldier and was followed by 'a very fine, if subdued rendering of the Soldier's Song, and then a beautiful playing of the Marseillaise'.

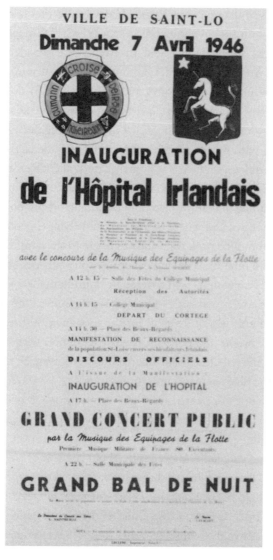

Poster for the inauguration ceremony of the Irish Hospital in Saint-Lô (courtesy Miss M. Crowley).

After speeches and music the assemblage returned to the Hospital where 'the Band played a short fanfare while the green, white and orange was slowly run up a huge flagstaff in a high position in the grounds – half way up our anthem was played, followed by the Marseillaise, arms presented by the gendarmes and a movie camera turning'. The remainder of the festive day was given over to an inspection of the hospital, with the provision of liberal hospitality, an open-air concert, a Ball in the town, and a smaller dance in the recreation hut of the hospital, which ended in the small hours of the morning. Patrick Carey recalls that many of the French, being unfamiliar with Irish whiskey, failed to see the day through.

The completed hospital consisted of twenty-five wooden huts, with the kitchen, theatres, X-ray department, treatment centres and wards concentrated in sixteen one-storey huts radiating from a main connecting corridor. The outpatients' department, casualty, laboratory, staff quarters, and two tubercular wards of twenty beds, the offices, stores and chapel occupied the remaining huts. The grounds were tastefully laid out with flowers, shrubs and vegetable gardens. According to Miss Crowley, 'the general appearance was homely, bright and cheerful, and besides the constant stream of patients, their relatives and friends, no stranger, I think, ever passed without calling and all received the hospitality of the house'. The hospital had an active maternity unit where the 'comfortable lying-in beds, with the swing cots attached, and mobile back rests added greatly to the comfort of the mothers and attracted much interest'. The surgical unit with twenty-six beds had a modern well-equipped theatre with its wall covered in aluminium plate and its floors with cork lino. With frequent casualties from exploding mines, the theatre was kept busy. The medical unit was in demand for the treatment of diseases of malnutrition. There was a bright and cheerful paediatric section with ten cots and two small side wards. The patients in the tuberculosis wards were all male, most of who had contracted the disease in concentration camps.

Many of the illnesses treated were due to malnutrition and neglect. Patrick Carey recalls two surgical operations, which, though minor, earned him lasting gratitude. A middle-aged peasant came to outpatients with the largest sebaceous cyst that the young surgeon had ever seen; about the size of a melon, it sprouted from his forehead like a second head that he was forced to support with his hands so that he could hold his head up; the misery of years of carrying this mill-stone was relieved by a brief operation. The Chief of the Gendarmerie in Saint-Lô had lost his son tragically in the bombing of the city, and his teenage daughter had had her leg amputated; his wife and he decided to have another child, and this belated arrival was brought to the Irish Hospital after drinking boiling liquid that caused life-threatening oedema of the glottis; death was only prevented by an emergency tracheostomy performed by Paddy Carey.

The hospital ambulance service, with its seven ambulances operating through -out the Normandy area, was much in demand. The wards filled up very quickly and with the gracious welcome afforded by the Irish, the queues for consultation grew daily, and one found there people worthy of admission to the court of mira- cles. The Irish welcomed everyone, so much so that a good woman, imagining herself ill despite the assurances of her doctor who steadfastly refused to send her to the hospital, declared: 'If that is all you can do, I will call the Irish and I tell you they will come and collect me in their ambulance if I call them, and they will do all that I ask of them.' What more beautiful tribute can be made?

General labour for the hospital was hard to come by and the French authori- ties provided thirteen German prisoners of war who were brought in each morning under armed guard and taken away in like fashion each evening, Miss Crowley found them 'well disciplined, always cheerful and willing to learn and the service they rendered played no small part in the success of the hospital'. She remembers her thirteen prisoners with affection, as they remember her and she still receives correspondence from some of those who survive. The prisoners were delivered to the hospital each morning by a French officer, and Miss Crowley immediately restored their dignity by replacing their prisoner-of-war garb with the uniforms of an orderly. None ever attempted to escape and Miss Crowley went so far as to take her clutch to the beaches of Normandy on picnics without a guard! Dr J. Gaffney also wrote warmly of the German POWs, who performed odd jobs for the staff: 'For example, they clean our shoes, brush our clothes, etc. and I have one whole-time in my lab, who is very useful at washing bottles, keeping an eye on my water-distillation plant and so forth.' The POW camp in Saint-Lô held about 1000 prisoners, among them being a doctor – Dr Lippit from Giaz, Austria – who had 'written to his people 84 times without getting a reply'.

Patrick Carey recalls that one of the German POWs fell on his bayonet prior to his capture, and the tip broke off, lodging in his buttock. The wound became infected and the prisoner seriously ill. Carey located the metal tip and successfully performed a difficult operation to remove it. On presenting the offending piece of weaponry proudly to his patient, he was somewhat taken aback when instead of an expression of gratitude, he was informed that had a German not invented X-rays, he would have been unable to locate it.

On 10 June 1946 Samuel Beckett, the storekeeper of Saint-Lô, wrote an account of the Irish Hospital for broadcasting to the Irish people on Radió Éireann. It is not known if this remarkable description of the Irish achievement in Saint-Lô was ever broadcast:

> On what a year ago was a grass slope, lying in the angle that the Vire and Bayeux roads make as they unite at the entrance of the town, opposite what remains of the second most important stud-farm in France, a general hospital now stands. It is the Hospital of the Irish Red Cross in Saint-Lô, or, as the Laudiniens themselves say, the Irish Hospital. The buildings consist of some 25 prefabricated wooden huts. They are superior, generally speaking, to those so scantily available for the wealthier, the better-connected, the astuter or the more flagrantly deserving of the bombed-out. Their finish, as well without as within, is the best that priority can command. They are lined with glass-wool and panelled in isorel, a strange substance of which only very limited supplies are available. There is real glass in the windows. The consequent atmosphere is that of brightness and airiness so comforting to sick people, and to weary staffs. The floors, where the exigencies of hygiene are greatest, are covered with linoleum. There was not enough linoleum left in France to do more than this. The walls and ceiling of the operating theatre are sheeted in aluminium of aeronautic origin, a decorative and practical solution of an old problem and a pleasant variation on the sword and ploughshare metamorphosis. A system of covered ways connects the kitchen with refectories and wards. The supply of electric current, for purposes both of heat and of power, leaves nothing to be desired. The hospital is centrally heated throughout, by means of coke. The medical, scientific, nursing and secretarial staffs are Irish, the instruments and furniture (including of course beds and bedding), the drugs and food, are supplied by the Society. I think I am right in saying that the number of in-patients (mixed) is in the neighbourhood of 90. As for the others, it is a regular thing, according to recent reports, for as many as 200 to be seen in the out-patients department in a day. Among such ambulant cases a large number are suffering from scabies and other diseases of the skin, the result no doubt of malnutrition or an ill-advised diet. Accident cases are frequent. Masonry falls when least expected, children play with detonators and demining continues. The laboratory, magnificently equipped, bids well to become the official laboratory for the department, if not of an even wider area. Considerable work has already been done in the analysis of local waters.

> These few facts, chosen not quite at random, are no doubt familiar already to those at all interested in the subject, and perhaps even to those of you listening to me now.

> They may not appear the most immediately instructive. That the operating-theatre should be sheeted with an expensive metal, or the floor of the labour-room covered with linoleum, can hardly be expected to interest those accustomed to such conditions as the sine qua non of reputable obstetrical

and surgical statistics. These are the sensible people who would rather have news of the Norman's semi-circular canals or resistance to sulphur than of his attitude to the Irish bringing gifts, who would prefer the history of our difficulties with an unfamiliar pharmacopeia and system of mensuration to the story of our dealings with the rare and famous ways of spirit that are the French ways. And yet the whole enterprise turned from the beginning on the establishing of a relation in the light of which the therapeutic relation faded to the merest of pretexts. What was important was not our having penicillin when they had none, nor the unregarding munificence of the French Ministry of Reconstruction (as it was then called), but the occasional glimpse obtained, by us in them and, who knows, by them in us (for they are an imaginative people), of that smile at the human condition as little to be extinguished by bombs as to be broadened by the elixirs of Burroughes and Welcome, the smile deriding, among other things, the having and not having, the giving and the taking, sickness and health.

It would not be seemly, in a retiring and indeed retired store-keeper, to describe the obstacles encountered in this connexion, and the forms, often grotesque, devised for them by the combined energies of the home and visiting temperaments. It must be supposed that they were not insurmountable, since they have long ceased to be of much account. When I reflect now on the recurrent problems of what, with all proper modesty, might be called the heroic period, on one in particular so arduous and elusive that it literally ceased to be formulable, I suspect that our pains were those inherent in the simple and necessary and yet so unattainable proposition that their way of being we, was not our way and that our way of being they, was not their way. It is only fair to say that many of us had never been abroad before.

Saint-Lô was bombed out of existence in one night. German prisoners of war, and casual labourers attracted by the relative food-plenty, but soon discouraged by housing conditions, continued, two years after the liberation, to clear away the debris, literally by hand. Their spirit has yet to learn the blessings of Gallup and their flesh the benefits of the bulldozer. One may thus be excused if one questions the opinion generally received, that ten years will be sufficient for the total reconstruction of Saint-Lô. But no matter what period of time must still be endured, before the town begins to resemble the pleasant and prosperous administrative and agricultural centre that it was, the hospital of wooden huts in its gardens between the Vire and Bayeux roads will continue to discharge its function, and its cured. 'Provisional' is not the term it was, in this universe become provisional. It will continue to discharge its function long after the Irish are gone and their names forgotten. But I think that to the end of its hospital days it will be called the Irish Hospital, and after that the huts, when they have been turned into dwellings, the Irish huts. I mention this possibility, in the hope that it will give general satisfaction. And having done so I may perhaps venture to mention another, more remote but perhaps of greater import in certain quarters, I mean the possibility that some of those who were in Saint-Lô will come home realising that they got at least as good as they gave, that they got indeed what they could hardly give, a vision and sense of a time-honoured conception of humanity in ruins, and perhaps even an inkling of the terms in which our condition is to be thought again.

These will have been in France.

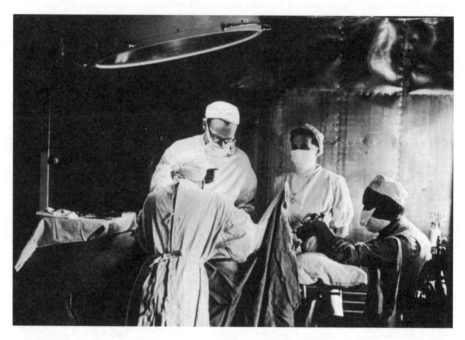

The operating theatre: Mr F. McKee is operating with Dr T. Boland giving the anaesthetic. Sister B. O'Rahilly is facing the camera and Sister M. Doherty has her back to the camera (courtesy Mr and Mrs P. Carey).

Such indeed was the case, as Dr Gaffney was to write: 'Looking up at the date I find it two months since I came here; and I must add that I've learned more about humanity and human nature in these two months than I'd learn at home in two years.' Colonel McKinney expressed similar sentiments:

We Irish doctors, and nurses have had the advantage of mixing closely with the French people, and we have been received warmly by many French families. We have learned more from this experience than would have been possible through many years of academic and touristic relations. We have seen the reaction of the people of France in its time of trial, and we have come to love and admire them. I regret departing this land to which I have been so attracted, but in so doing I express for my colleagues and myself, our respect for this noble country. I pay homage to the greatness of France and the courage of its people.

Beckett's broadcast is of interest in that it gives not only an account of the Irish Hospital, but describes also the emotional consequences of the experience, or, at least, what the enduring feelings were for one of his sensitivity. Beckett expresses emotion most deeply in poetry and two profound poems emanate from his experiences and a friendship in Saint-Lô. The first, entitled simply 'Saint-Lô', was published in *The Irish Times* on 24 June 1946. It is a complex statement on the survival of humanity in the depth of ruin and despair and is generally regarded as one of his finest poems. The river Vire winding its way through the ruined city links the past, the destruction of the present, and the inevitable rebirth witnessed by Beckett, with the havoc that all-forgetting humanity will just as inevitably inflict upon itself again:

> Vire will wind in other shadows
> unborn through the bright ways tremble
> and the old mind ghost-forsaken
> sink into its havoc

Arthur Darley contracted tuberculosis either at Saint-Lô, where he was in charge of the tuberculosis unit, or shortly before his departure from Ireland to serve with the Red Cross. Fluent in French, gentle in manner, and selfless in his dedication to the sick of Saint-Lô, he was most popular with the patients. He began his outpatients clinic (for which patients began queuing before dawn) at 9 AM and continued through the day to 6 PM. Appreciation was shown by gifts of Calvados of which Darley had an immense stock. This he indulged in occasionally himself, always placing his violin in the safekeeping of Miss Crowley, before an evening in the town. His death in 1948 distressed Beckett deeply and he wrote the poem 'Mort de A.D'. in tribute to his friend. In this poem (which Beckett never translated, but which is translated here by Edith Fournier), he expressed his anguish at his friend's suffering, the futility of existence destined to pain before annihilation, and the spiritual hunger of Darley, eased only by his frantic reading of the 'lives of the saints':

> and to be there still there
> clinging to my old poxed board of blackness
> days and nights milled blindfold
> to be there not fleeing and to flee and to be there
> stooping towards time in throes that owns

to having been what it was done what it did
of me of my friend who died yesterday gleam eyed
long toothed panting in his beard devouring
the lives of saints a life a day's life
living his dark sins over again at night
yesterday dead whilst I was drawing breath
and to be there draining high up above the storm
the dregs of irretrievable time
clutching the old slat a witness to departures
a witness to home-comings

Beckett's last task at Saint-Lô was to obtain rat poison from Paris to enable the matron, Mary Crowley, to rid the maternity and children's wards of infestation. His resignation was effective from January 1946, but he continued to give whatever help he could to the hospital from Paris.

And what of this remarkable institution, the Hôpital Irlandais de Saint-Lô? On 31 December 1946 it was handed over to the French Red Cross as a fully functioning hospital, which later was rebuilt and is now a major hospital in the town. The citizens of Saint-Lô demonstrated their appreciation to the Irish staff on their departure, when it is recorded that 'the entire population [...] headed by the Mayor, and crowds from other parts of Normandy, marched to the Hospital with banners bearing words of appreciation, presented floral tributes to and warmly acclaimed the departing staff'. There were many tributes:

> Ireland and her Red Cross (which was only founded in 1939) are well deserving of the gratitude of the Normands, who were the first to receive the beneficence of this organisation. The Irish Hospital not only welcomed the sick, it also received the curious like me, and it was while toasting the whiskey, 'the Calva', of Ireland, that I made acquaintance with these admirable people whom we adopted and received so gratefully within our walls – our walls which exist no more.

The French government expressed its gratitude to the Irish staff of the Hôpital De La Croix Rouge Irlandaise with the award of the Medaille de la Reconnaissance Française. Dr Alan Thompson returned to his post of senior physician on the staff of the Richmond Hospital in Dublin. He was appointed professor of medicine to the Royal College of Surgeons in Ireland in 1962. His distinguished position in Dublin medicine was acknowledged by his profession when he was elected to the office of president of the Royal College of Physicians of Ireland in 1966, and in 1967 when the College celebrated its tercentenary. Alan Thompson died on 23 March 1974.

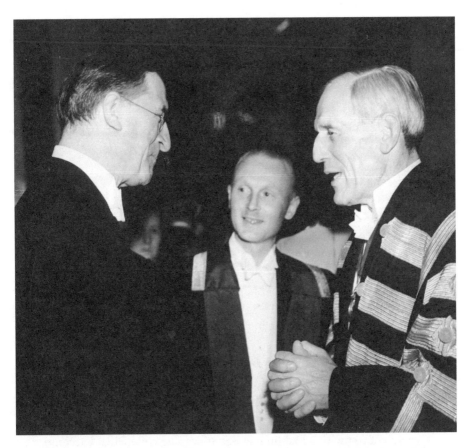

Alan Thompson (centre) *with Éamon de Valera, President of Ireland* (to his right),
and Bethel Solomons, president of the Royal College of Physicians of Ireland, 1946–8
(The Irish Times *photograph, courtesy the Royal College of Physicians of Ireland).*

Arthur Darley died from tuberculosis at Our Lady's Hospice, Harold's Cross, on 30 December 1948. He had revisited Saint-Lô shortly before his death.

James Gaffney returned to Sir Patrick Dun's Hospital. He was killed tragically in the Aer Lingus aeroplane crash in the Welsh mountains on 10 January 1952.

Miss Mary Crowley returned to Dublin where she played an active role in the development of nursing, becoming the founder dean of the Faculty of Nursing of the Royal College of Surgeons in Ireland. She died in March 1990.

Samuel Beckett continued to live in Paris where he died on 22 December 1989. He was awarded the Nobel Prize for literature in 1969 for 'a body of work that, in new forms of fiction and the theatre, has transmuted the destitution of modern man into his exaltation'.

A.J. (Con) Leventhal

THE JEWISH COMMUNITY in Dublin brought much to the city – industry, culture, character – and above all humour. All of these characteristics are embodied in the fictional Bloom of *Ulysses* but they were also to be found in the persona of A.J. (Con) Leventhal.

My first contact with a Dublin Jew was as a young child when I accompanied my father to Ballybrack to visit his friend Bethel Solomons, a renowned Dublin figure, who became the first Jewish master of the Rotunda Hospital from 1926 to 1933, earned ten international rugby caps for his country between 1908 and 1910 and served as president of the Royal College of Physicians of Ireland from 1946 to 1948. My memories of this occasion is of a strikingly handsome man taking me by the hand down the long garden to his summer house where he was writing his autobiography, *One Doctor in His Time*, which was published in 1956.

My next contact with Dublin Judaism was to endure due to the curious vagaries of what we call destiny. I became ill with tuberculosis when a young schoolboy and was confined to house if not bed for some nine months. My father, whose speciality in medicine was tuberculosis, did not however treat me in keeping with best practice and called in his colleague and friend Leonard Abrahamson, who was professor of medicine at the Royal College of Surgeons and senior physician (with my father and Alan Thompson) at the Richmond Hospital. My earliest memories of Professor Abrahamson are of a kind and gentle man whose presence was announced by the smell of cigar smoke wafting up the stairs to my bedroom ahead of his appearance. Later, much later, I succeeded his son Meryvn (Muff) as acting professor of Materia Medica and Therapeutics at the Royal College of Surgeons in Ireland, when he departed Ireland to work in Israel in 1973. I then inherited Muff's Jewish practice and so came into contact with a diverse gathering of Dublin Jews and learned to admire their individuality even to an outsider, I could not fathom their religion and customs. When I worked in general practice in Smethwick in Birmingham – an eye-opener for a sheltered youth from Dublin, where the election slogans read: 'If you want a Nigger for a neighbour, vote Labour' – Tona and I befriended another delightful Jewish couple late of Dublin, Ivor and Phyllis Radnor. Then came Con Leventhal, sometime in the seventies, epitomizing all that had made Joyce choose a Dublin Jew for the heroic role in *Ulysses*.

Con had succeeded Samuel Beckett at Trinity College as lecturer in English and French in 1932. In 1958 he married Ethna McCarthy on the death of his first wife, and when Ethna died in 1961, he married Marion Leigh. He retired to Paris in 1963 to join his friend Samuel Beckett. These sparse details ignore what can never be done justice in words, what can never be known in its fullness, namely the patient intellect that was able to enhance the expression of a greater talent, maybe sublimating itself in so doing. Con also threw a protective mantle around his friend, besieged, as he was, by so many admirers.

Con and Marion were regular visitors to our home when they came to Dublin from Paris, and I visited them in their book-lined flat on boulevard Montparnasse whenever I went to Paris from where we would go to La Coupole across the road and dine late into the night. When Con became ill in 1979 I accompanied him from Dublin to boulevard Montparnasse, where he died shortly afterwards. It is fair to say, I think, that from having been a dominant intellectual figure in Dublin from the 1930s to the 1960s, he was almost forgotten at the time of his death and even in his alma mater Trinity College where, to use an Irish expression, 'He had once been a power in the land', he was but little known. I determined that he should not pass into the mists of posterity unheeded. Two years after his death I brought together a band of loyal friends (that included Samuel Beckett) 'to consider how best to commemorate his erudition, charm and literary influence'. It was resolved to establish a scholarship that would enable an Irish graduate student in English or Modern Languages of Trinity College, Dubli,n to study in Europe. Con's friends and literary associates, and academic institutes at home and abroad contributed generously to the scholarship fund and to the scholarship auction in the Samuel Beckett Rooms in Trinity College on 15 March 1984. The inaugural Leventhal scholarship was awarded to Alan Gilsenan, who has made a number of award-winning documentaries, and is presently Chairperson of the Irish Film Institute, and the scholarship has been awarded annually since then.

The essay on Con Leventhal is based on 'From the Waters of Zion to Liffey-side', the Leonard Abrahamson Memorial Lecture that I delivered in the Royal College of Surgeons in Ireland in 1981[6] in which I attempted to outline the remark-able contribution of the Jewish diaspora to Ireland, and in particular to the city of Dublin, and on 'The Writings of A.J. Leventhal', a brief biographical summary of Leventhal's literary achievements, which was written in 1984 for *A.J. Leventhal 1896–1979. Dublin Scholar, Wit and Man of Letters*, to highlight the establishment of the Leventhal Scholarship in Trinity College, Dublin.[7]

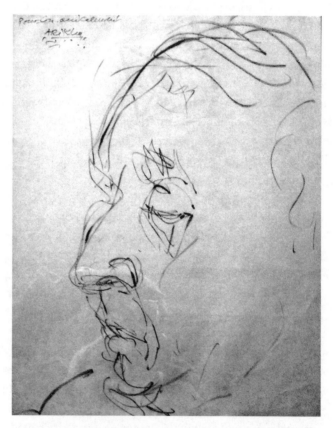

Con Leventhal sketched by Avigdor Arikha in a Parisian café.

From the Waters of Zion to Liffeyside, 1981

THE WARS of upheaval in eighteenth-century Europe drove many poor Jews from Germany and Poland to London and hence to Dublin, but unrest and uncertainty in Ireland caused many of the wealthy Sephardi to depart back to England or onwards to the New World. Towards the close of the century the Jewish community was in a precarious state. Most of the wealthy Sephardi had left, and the poorer Ashkenazi had difficulty in sustaining the community.

With the right of naturalization Polish and German Jews from England came to settle in Dublin. Then in 1881 the May Laws were introduced in Russia, and there began the great influx of Lithuanian Jews to the city. In 1881 the Dublin Jewish community numbered only 300 whereas at the turn of the century there were 2000.

The Dublin Jew, with his multi-racial background and Judaic philosophy, intrigued, amused, at times irritated, but in the end influenced greatly the Irish character of the Dubliner. And the Jew in his turn blended into the character of the city to the extent of remaining individual but being unmistakably a Dubliner. All Dubliners absorb in their development something of the Jewish tradition, and although not all are aware of the extent of the Jewish influence, few can fail to notice its presence. One departed Dubliner, James Joyce, who was unable to forget the city simply because he was determined to recreate it, and who was more aware than most of the Jewish influence, took with him the embryonic concept that was to become Leopold Bloom, one of literature's most celebrated Jews.

Joyce's Jew, Leopold Bloom, is an in-depth portrayal of the Dublin Jew at the turn of the century. Bloom's father Rudolph Virag, a Hungarian Jew from Szombathely, Vienna, Budapest, Milan and London was converted from the Israelite faith to Protestantism by the Society for Promoting Christianity among the Jews, and died by his own hand in Ennis. The son, Leopold Bloom, was baptized no less than three times – first in the protestant church of St Nicolas Without, then under a pump in the village of Swords, and finally as a Catholic by the Reverend Malone in the church of the Three Patrons in Rathgar before his marriage to Molly. Although ostensibly a Catholic, Bloom was at heart a Jew. Why then did Joyce make him a Catholic? Historically as we have seen there were good reasons but that is not enough. Bloom's Catholicism permits us to look through Bloom's eye – a very jaundiced one – at his adopted religion:

> Good idea the Latin. Stupefies them first ... Then feel like one family party, same in the theatre, all in the same swim ... Not so lonely ... Those

THE WEIGHT OF COMPASSION & OTHER ESSAYS

crawthumpers, now that's a good name for them, there's always something shifty looking about them. They're not straight men of business either ... Wonderful organisation certainly, goes like clockwork. Confession ... Great weapon in their hands. More than doctor or solicitor ... Squareheaded chaps those must be in Rome: they work the whole show. And don't they rake in the money too?

How effectively Joyce removes himself from invective by letting the Jew, one of a foreign religion and yet a convert and therefore *au fait* with the teachings of Rome, give free rein to his thoughts on those ministers of Catholicism of whom Joyce was so critical: 'Eat you out of house and home. No families themselves to feed. Living on the fat of the land. Their butteries and larders. I'd like to see them do the black fast of Yom Kippur.' What a melange of Jewish humour and Dublin wit and Joycean genius there is in Bloom's one-sentenced analysis of nuns: 'It was a nun they say invented barbed wire.'

What anti-Semitism there is in *Ulysses* is comparatively mild, but it was palpable in Dublin at the turn of the century and Joyce did not fail to observe it. In fact it serves his purpose very well – what better foil for the injustices and hypocrisy of Catholicism than Dublin anti-Semitism, and what better target than the gentle, humorous, sensitive character that is Bloom? But Bloom serves Joyce further as a means of exposing the futility of anti-Semitism, although he is unable to explain its irrationality: 'When in doubt persecute Bloom.' Deasy explains to young Stephen Dedalus that 'England is in the hand of the jews. In all the highest places: her finance, her press. And they are the signs of a nation's decay ... As sure as we are standing here the jew merchants are already at their work of destruction. Old England is dying.' But, asks Stephen, 'is not a merchant one who buys cheap and sells dear, be he jew or gentile?' In the hospitable ambience of Barney Kiernan's public house at numbers 9, 10 and 11 Little Britain Street we are given one of the great moments of Joycean epiphany and Dublin anti-Semitism. What better fuse for the bang than alcohol, and what better flame than that favoured topic of Irish pub conversation – God, or his immediate descendants and close relatives. Bloom, accustomed to mild taunts from the drinking Dubliners, ignores the likes of 'We want no more strangers in our house', but is finally goaded to retribution by a slur on his nationality. He declares, 'Mendelssohn was a jew and Karl Marx and Mercadante and Spinoza. And the Saviour was a jew ... Your God was a jew. Christ was a jew like me.' This blasphemy, for such it is taken to be, provokes an immediate reaction: 'By Jesus ... I'll brain that bloody jewman for using the holy name. By Jesus, I'll crucify him so I will.' And with what does the noble citizen

endeavour to give to Dublin that which it would so dearly like – a real live cruci-
fixion? With a biscuit tin hurled after Bloom as he canters down the Liffeyside
in a jaunting car. Later Bloom reflects on his victory and concludes that the truth
has been particularly shocking for the gathering 'because mostly they appeared to
imagine that he [God] came from Carrick-on-Shannon or somewhere about in
the county Sligo'.

Bloom is handsome; Bloom is libidinous, and women find Bloom agreeable.
Bloom is kind to his fellow Dubliners and to animals; Bloom is cultured – as
Lenehen remarks to McCoy on Wellington Quay – 'he's a cultured allroundman.
Bloom is he's not one of your common or garden … you know … There's a touch
of the artist about old Bloom.' This is important to Joyce's theme; he regards
Jewish culture as superior to most – 'The Jews in the wilderness and on the mountain top said, *It is meet to be here. Let us build an altar to Jehovah.* The Roman in
the same situation said – *It is meet to be here: Let us construct a water-closet.*' Bloom
loves music; Bloom is a diplomat and a gentleman; Bloom is a man of only modest
means; Bloom is a freemason. Bloom is temperate – almost a complete TT as
Davy Byrne was to remark to Nosey Flynn – 'I often saw him in here and I never
once saw him, you know, over the line.' Bloom's abstemiousness is in contrast to
his gentile fellow Dubliner. Again we have an example of Joyce using Bloom to
illuminate aspects of character peculiar to the Irish: 'Ireland sober is Ireland free.'
Bloom is Irish and proud to be: 'What is your nation if I may ask, says the citizen
– Ireland, says Bloom. I was born here. Ireland.' We know that Joyce was fond of
Jews, but he was often irritated and bored by them, and Bloom is a bloody bore:
'I declare to my antimacassar if you took up a straw from the bloody floor and if
you said to Bloom: *Look at, Bloom. Do you see that straw? That's a straw.* Declare to
my aunt he'd talk about it for an hour so he would and talk steady.' On another
occasion, Stephen unable to stand Bloom's dissertation on Ireland any longer says,
'We can't change the country. Let us change the subject.'

But of all Bloom's traits, it is the wanderer and the exile in him that appeals
most to Joyce. Bloom is neither accepted nor rejected by Dublin. He is never
completely at home, because he has no home. To add to his isolation he has left
his religion, and is no longer accepted by his own people. Though Bloom is exiled,
he accepts his lot without much difficulty, and at heart likes Dublin. He fanta-
sizes about travel and Zion, but he can never bring himself to do anything about
either. Joyce identifies readily with the exiled spirit. Like the Jew he knows the
call of the homeland: 'They have forgotten Kevin Egan, not he them. Remem-
bering thee, O Sion.'

The Jew, the diaspora, the distillation of centuries, the instillation of diverse cultures, and for all their differences the blending of Irish and Jewish cultures and their mutual, albeit begrudging, admiration for each other is what makes Bloom the Dublin Jew, the everyman of all men's philosophy: 'The oldest people. Wandered far away over all the earth, captivity to captivity, multiplying, dying, being born everywhere.' How like the Jews were the Irish once – invaded, persecuted, decimated by the famine, exiled and dispersed to foreign lands, to 'the greater Ireland beyond the sea'.

The similarities were seen thus by Joyce in 1904:

> The presence of guttural sounds, diacritic aspirations, epenthetic and servile letters in both languages: their antiquity, both having been taught on the plain of Shinar 242 years after the deluge in the seminary instituted by Fenius Farsaigh, descendant of Noah, progenitor of Israel, and ascendant of Heber and Heremon progenitors of Ireland: their archaeological, genealogical, hagiographical, exegetical, homilectic, toponomastic, historical and religious literatures comprising the works of rabbis and culdees, Torah, Talmud (Mischana and Ghemara) Massor, Pentateuch, Book of the Dun Cow, Book of Ballymote, Garland of Howth, Book of Kells: their dispersal, persecution, survival and revival: the isolation of their synagogical and ecclesiastical rites in ghetto (S. Mary's Abbey) and masshouse (Adam and Eves' tavern): The proscription of their national costumes in penal laws and jewish dress acts: the restoration in Chanan David of Zion and the possibility of Irish political autonomy or devolution.

Let us bestir ourselves from *Ulysses* – 'An epic of two races (Israelite-Irish) and at the same time the cycle of the human body, as well as a little story of a day (life).' 'Old Methusalem Bloom' embodies all the weaknesses and the strengths, the humour and the sadness, the myth and the reality, the past and the future dreams, that was the Dublin Jew at the turn of the century. Let us look now at the dream become reality.

The first signs of Jewish intellectual development in the twentieth century were to be seen in a remarkable group of young Jews at Trinity College. To name but a few there was Bethel Solomons, Leonard Abrahamson, A.J. Leventhal, Eddie Lippmann and Michael Noyek.

At this time there lived at 32 Waterloo Road an exemplary Jewish couple, Maurice and Rosa Solomons. Maurice, born in Dublin of English parents, was an Imperialist who claimed Irish Nationality. A successful optician who wrote some dramatic criticism, he was a student of free-masonry and was successful in a number of businesses. He was honorary consul in Dublin to the old Austro-Hungarian

Empire. His wife Rosa from Yorkshire was an imaginative and cultured woman who wrote pleasant verse, spoke many languages and was an accomplished musician. Active in Jewish community affairs, she was one of the driving forces in the establishment of the Synagogue at Adelaide Road. Together, she and her husband founded the first secular school for Jewish children in Dublin. One of their four children Bethel was educated at St Andrew's School, where he showed academic promise and aptitude for sport, particularly rugby. His father, who had himself aspired towards medicine, sent his son to Trinity, where as a medical student he excelled in rugby and captained the first fifteen. At Sir Patrick Duns Hospital he walked the wards, but found ample time to relax with Guinness available at one shilling and ten pence per dozen, whiskey at two and a half pence a glass, and pipe tobacco to be had for five pence an ounce. Bethel was very close to his younger sister Estella, and she was able to introduce the medical student to the artistic and literary youth of the city.

Estella had been educated firstly at Miss Wade's School for Young Ladies on Morehampton Road, then in Hanover where she became fluent in German, and finally at Alexandra College. She went from there to the Dublin Metropolitan School of Art. A bewitchingly beautiful girl, with sensuous eyes and a gypsy-like expression (as her later self-portrait shows), she had a sensitive and sweet personality that endeared her to all. At the Metropolitan School one of her teachers was William Orpen and she later went to the school that he and Augustus John (Æ) opened in London and there she was to be greatly influenced by Walter Osborne. At this early stage she excelled in etching, and the magic of her Dublin street scenes is to be seen in Kelleher's *The Glamour of Dublin* and other books that she illustrated.

Two other bright Jewish children entered Trinity together in the early twentieth century to study modern languages. They were Leonard Abrahamson and Abraham Jacob Leventhal, known affectionately to his friends as Con. Outwardly he had the appurtenances of a serious boy but he was full of humour, and passionately fond of books and literature. He entered Trinity with a Board Examination and completed his course with the degree of Senior Moderator and later he was awarded his doctorate in Philosophy. He wrote with humour, affection and some sadness about Jewish Dublin in the early part of this century.

> When I look back on those days it seems to me that we young jewish boys must have appeared curious creatures to our young native neighbours. Though we attended the same National Schools, played the same games, spoke the same language and returned to our dinners at the same hour yet there were definite differences. We looked foreign, to begin with. And

in the afternoons when all schoolboys left their homes to indulge in such street games as marbles, relievo, handball and the like, we were not available. Secular schooling for the day was over but we had still to spend a further two to three hours at Hebrew school.

The young Jewish schoolboy in Dublin did not have it easy, but he learned to give as good as he got both in pugilism and wit. The Lombard Street Catholics had for their battle cry a verse that went as follows:

> 'Two shillies, two shillies,' the jewman did cry,
> For a fine pair of blankets from me you did buy;
> Do you think me von idjit or von bloomin' fool,
> If I don't get my shillie I must have my vool.

How quickly the young Oakfield Israelites capitalized on the great weakness of their taunters with:

> 'Two pennies, two pennies', the Christian did shout,
> 'For a bottle of porter or Guinness's stout;
> My wife's got no shawl and my kids have no shoes,
> But I must have my money. I must have my booze.'

Much of the difference between the Jew and his fellow Dubliner was one of creed rather than race, or as Con Leventhal puts it, 'Thus, while the Sassenach might have referred to the drunken Irish, we merely saw tippling followers of Christ.'

Leonard Abrahamson was born a few years before the turn of the century in Russia and the family then immigrated to Ireland and settled in Newry where Leonard was sent to the Christian Brothers School. He entered Trinity College in 1912 with an entrance prize in Hebrew and modern Irish, and was awarded a Sizarship in Irish. With Con Leventhal he studied French and German, and obtained first-class honours in all examinations for three successive years. He was an active member of the Dublin Union Gaelic Society and represented Trinity in the Intervarsity Debates that were held in Irish. This Society's activities were suspended when its members ignored the Provost's opposition and invited Padraig Pearse to address them. Leonard was awarded a Foundation Scholarship in Modern Languages and was a Senior Exhibitioner.

However he decided that medicine rather than arts was to be his career, and he proved no less successful in this course of study. He obtained first-class honours in Midwifery, Surgery and Medicine, won the FitzPatrick Prize and was awarded the University Travelling Prize in Medicine. In 1919 he married Tillie Nurock and went to Paris for a year's postgraduate study.

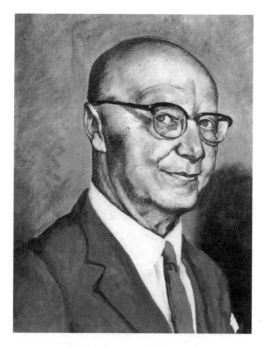

*Leonard Abrahamson by Harry Kernoff. Portrait
in the Royal College of Surgeons in Ireland.*

Two other students not disinterested in politics were Eddie Lippman, a medical student, and Michael Noyek, who had a distinguished academic career at Trinity. He became much involved in the politics of the day and was later to become famous for his defence of many Sinn Féin Nationalists, and was to be close friend and legal adviser to Michael Collins. The political happenings of a country about to demand its freedom were not passing unnoticed by the Jewish community outside the University. Many a young Dublin Jew found himself torn between two loyalties. Patriotically he aligned himself with the country of his birth or adoption, whilst at the same time being conscious of his own race and religion. The Jew's loyalty to his adopted nation may be very intense and none was to demonstrate this more selflessly than a young Jewish boy brought up in an apartment above a furniture shop on the Liffeyside.

Robert Briscoe, born in 1894, learned from his Lithuanian father Abraham about Wolfe Tone, Robert Emmet and Charles Stewart Parnell at an early age. As a young boy he had watched Queen Victoria's procession to Dublin from Kings-town. Later, as a prospecting young business man in America he heard with horror of the Easter Executions, and returned to Dublin with Liam Mellows having sold his business interests. In Dublin he joined the IRA and gave himself totally to their cause. He was much influenced by de Valera whom he saw as one having 'the indomitable determination of a Washington; the militant faith of St Paul and the moral grandeur of the Prophet Elija'. A peaceful, rather humble, Jewish wool merchant with a knowledge of the German language and German business methods was ideally suited for gun-running missions between Ireland and the Continent, a hazardous occupation that young Briscoe accomplished successfully for many years.

Bethel Solomons, having graduated from Trinity and then studied for a time in Paris, was appointed assistant master at the Rotunda Hospital, where he began to turn his energies towards making obstetrics his career. To judge from his reminiscences of those days, student life in that Rabelaisian institute was little different from later years, although the nurses were unable to participate as freely. It was looked upon as a most serious misdemeanour when a group of final-year students in drunken unison sang outside the matron's door, 'We want hot buttered nurses on toast.'

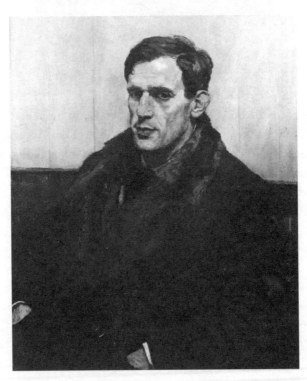

Bethel Solomons painted by his sister Estella Solomons
(courtesy the late Michael Solomons).

Bethel did not devote himself entirely to medicine. He was capped ten times for playing rugby for Ireland, and was the first Jew to play for his country. There is the delightful mot of the Dublin wag who, being asked what he thought of Ireland's chances, replied, 'Ireland – you call that Ireland, fourteen Protestants and one bloody Jew.' He was the first Jew to become master of the Rotunda Hospital and to be elected president of the Royal College of Physicians in Ireland, an event that *The Irish Times* reported as follows: 'Dr Bethel Solmons who has been elected president of the Royal College of Physicians of Ireland, played rugby for Ireland ten times.' Proud to be a Jew he wrote thus: 'I do not think that there can ever be real converts from our ancient race. We are born Jews and nothing can alter that fact. Why a Jew would want to forsake his birthright is a mystery to me, for he can be very proud to belong to a people who have done so much for mankind.'

Bethel was a keen rider to hounds and one day an American visitor enquiring who he was was told, 'Oh, that's Dr Solomons, the master of the Rotunda.' 'What pack is that? I have never heard of it,' asked the American. 'It is one of the most notable packs in Ireland – the Maternity Harriers,' was the rejoinder. Successful in practice, handsome in appearance and attractive in manner, he was a well-known and respected figure in the city. With Estella he was part of the Dublin literary circle. James Stephens was a close friend and dedicated his first novel *The Charwoman's Daughter* to him, and Denis Johnston inscribed a play, 'To B.S. because of the part he took in my greatest work' – the birth of his children.

Estella was making quite a reputation as a painter. These were exciting times for an artist. In Dublin Jack Yeats was beginning to achieve recognition. No one did more to promote his reputation than Victor Waddington through his art galleries in Dublin and London. Then there was the influence of the Impressionist movement to which Estella was inevitably drawn. She was also attracted to politics with Kathleen Goodfellow, whose patriotic writings appeared under the pseudonym of Michael Scot. She enlisted in Cumann na mBan and thereafter Estella's studio at Great Brunswick Street became a place of refuge for those on the run. Estella was able to meet and paint portraits of Irish patriots and these have been collected in a small volume by Hilary Pyle. Estella married James Starkey, better known by his *nom de plume* of Seumas O'Sullivan. A tall handsome poet with a slight stoop, he carried a pipe and walking stick wherever he went. Actor, poet, publisher, bibliophile, he will probably be best remembered as the editor of the *Dublin Magazine*, which he founded in 1923 and brought out quarterly until publication ceased with his death in 1958.

His remarkable journal survived difficult times, and much of the credit for its success must go to Estella and Kathleen Goodfellow. When Con Leventhal submitted a review of *Ulysses* Leventhal had to found the little magazine named *The Klaxon*, which survived just long enough to publish his review under the pseudonym of L.K. Emery. At least the effort earned him the gratitude of Joyce for one of the most prescient criticisms of his novel. In the *Dublin Magazine* hitherto unknown and little published poets were launched in print – Patrick Kavanagh, Patrick McDonagh, Alun Lewis, Samuel Beckett and John Montague are examples of Seumas O'Sullivan's remarkable ability to recognize talent. Estella and Seumas lived at first in a large house called The Grange in Rathfarnham, where on Sunday afternoons and evenings after a prolonged and sumptuous tea, the collected literati would play croquet. Gogarty was probably responsible for the story of the rustic in the bus who pointed to The Grange and exclaimed to the passengers that the man who lived there was 'a jewman be the name of Seamus O'Soloman'.

The Starkey salon at The Grange and later at Morehampton Road included Æ, W.B. Yeats, Stephens, Leventhal, Austin Clark, Michael Noyek, Steven MacKenna, Cathal O'Shannon, Patrick McDonagh, Mary Lavin, Beatrice Gleneavy, Albert Power, and Niall Sheridan, whose imitation of Brinsley MacNamara was so good Seamus used to say that when he met Brinsley he got the impression that the latter was imitating Niall imitating himself. These were the halcyon days when Dublin was the largest village in Europe, and in this village another Jewish artist Harry Kernoff was endearing himself to the people with his paintings of Dublin scenery and its citizens.

If Leopold Bloom was the wandering Jew in mind, then Bob Briscoe was him in reality. When the Civil War broke out he was on the move again, this time to New York to further the Republican cause.

One way in which he did this was to take over the Irish Consular Offices in New York from the Free State government, and to proclaim them held for the Irish Republican government. The occupation, which did not last long, appears to have been managed with humour and tact on all sides, and was seen by the Americans as an event almost too Irish to be true, and furthermore taking place right in New York. Briscoe and his companions were finally lifted gently from the offices by the burly New York cops many of whom were Irish, on the directive of my grandfather, Professor Timothy Smiddy, who was Free State Minister Plenipotentiary to Washington, and as such was understandably anxious to reoccupy the Consular Offices.

In 1927 Briscoe was elected to the Dáil and he has left us some interesting vignettes of the 'Chief'. When Vladimir Jabotinsky came to Ireland to study IRA methods for his militant Zionist organization, the Irgun, Briscoe arranged for him to meet de Valera. 'How can the Jews establish a legitimate claim to Palestine?'

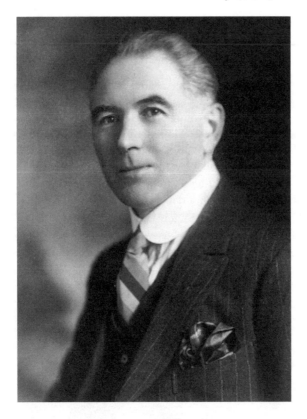

Timothy Smiddy.

asked Dev. 'Did they not leave it; and has it not been in the possession of the Arabs for nearly 2000 years?' Jabotinsky answered:

> Mr De Valera, I have been reading Irish history. As a result of the great famine of 1847 and 1848, I believe the population of Ireland fell from 8 millions to 4 millions. Now supposing it had been reduced to 50,000 and the country had been resettled by the Welsh, Scots and English, would you then have given up the claim of Ireland for the Irish?

In 1937 when the British government proposed to partition Palestine between Jews and Arabs, Professor Brodetsky came from England to see de Valera to persuade him to support partition when it came before the League of Nations.

De Valera replied:

> Professor, I read the Old Testament many years ago. I am afraid I have forgotten many things I read; but one passage I recall clearly. It is the story of Solomon's judgement of the two women who claimed the same baby. I

remember how when Solomon ruled that the baby be divided the real mother screamed. 'No! No! Give the baby to the other woman!' This is my answer to partition. The rightful owners of a country will never agree to partition.

In 1938 Briscoe was on the move again – this time to Warsaw to the Jewish ghettos. He described his meeting with the Chief Rabbi as follows:

The chief rabbi was a big man wearing a long black coat and a magnificent black beard. Glassy black side curls hung beneath his flat black hat. The other two rabbis were smaller but identical in their sombre garb. To these men then I made my plea that they consent to a plan for large-scale emigration to Palestine. I spoke with an ardour and eloquence inspired by the terrible urgency I felt … Standing like a figure carved in basalt on a Judean tomb, with Europe in flames around him and Azrael soaring on sable wings above his people, he gave this pronouncement, 'We must wait for the Messiah to lead us to the Holy Land. All forms of Zionism are to us *traif* (unclean).'

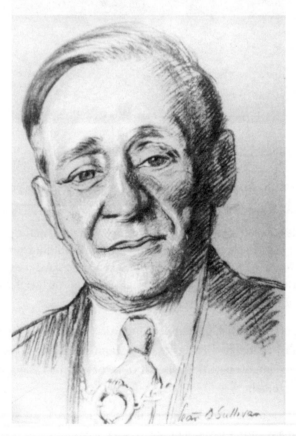

Robert Briscoe. Portrait by Sean O'Sullivan.

In 1956 Robert Briscoe was elected Lord Mayor of Dublin, a position to which no other Jew had risen. He was one of Dublin's most popular Lord Mayors, and when he died, the Americans, who idolized him, wanted to commemorate 'The Fabulous Irishman', as they called him, in a Broadway musical.

Many Dublin Jews moved between Dublin and other cities and some left Dublin altogether. To London went Hannah Berman; Hannah a member of the Zlotover family from Lithuania, left Dublin after the publication of her first novel *Meletovna* in 1914. She attempted to recreate the spirit of Yiddish folk writing in English, and was in the opinion of Con Leventhal a neglected Irish Jewish novelist. Hyman Edelstein, a classical scholar, a talented poet and prose writer, left Dublin to settle in Montreal. And that figure that has cropped up so much – Con Leventhal finally settled in Paris, where he continued his literary criticism. He will, I feel, come to be recognized as one of the great significant background figures of twentieth-century literature. Friend and adviser to Joyce and subsequently friend and confidant of Sam Beckett, he was the epitome of cultural sensitivity and sophistication.

Let us close by focusing our attention on Leonard Abrahamson – or the Abe as he was affectionately called. Appointed to Mercers Hospital in 1922 he was the first doctor in this country to study electrocardiography, then a new technique. He founded the first department of electrocardiography, which was subsequently taken over by another Jewish cardiologist of repute – Joe Lewis. From a study of the Abe's papers, it is clear that he had mastered the new innovation and saw clearly the great potential for its development in cardiology. He was appointed to the chair of pharmacology in 1926, became a member of the Richmond Hospital Staff in 1932, and a professor of medicine in the Royal College of Surgeons in 1934. He was president of the Royal College of Physicians of Ireland for three years, president of the Section of Medicine of the Royal Irish Academy, president of the Biological Society of Trinity College and the College of Surgeons, and a founder member of the British Cardiac Society. In addition to his medical activities, he was active in Jewish community work and was honorary president of the Jewish National Fund. But as I have said at the outset it was his humour, wit and ability to communicate as a lecturer that made him unique as a clinical teacher, and a character. 'There is only one thing,' he remarked, 'that I like writing better than a bill and that is a receipt.'

What a marvellous mixture of Jewish and Dublin humour and wit there is in the delightful Flood-Abrahamson clash that took place in the Academy of Medicine. J.C. Flood, surgeon to the Charitable Infirmary, Jervis Street, was renowned and feared as a wit and orator. In addition to his medical degree he had a Bachelor of Arts, a Bachelor of Commerce, and he was a Barrister at Law. He had also a postgraduate doctorate of medicine, and a Master's in Surgery. When he was later to give up medicine to join the Benedictine Order, he would acquire doctorates of canon law and moral theology in Rome. On the evening in question, the Abe presented to the Academy a complicated case of a woman with rheumatoid arthritis, to whom he had given gold injections over many years. Eventually after many remissions and relapses the patient succumbed to her illness and died. In his presentation Abe had clearly demonstrated the beneficial effect of gold. When the applause from the impressed and appreciative audience had ceased, Flood rose and asked if he might enquire from the learned professor if he had managed to recover the gold after the good lady's demise. *Touché* it seemed, but the Abe was to have the last laugh when he said, 'Flood has more degrees than a thermometer without the same capacity for registering warmth.'

The Writings of A.J. Leventhal, 1984

CON LEVENTHAL was born in Dublin in 1896, and educated at Wesley College. His childhood experiences in Catholic Dublin are recounted with humour and poignancy in 'What it means to be a Jew'. His undergraduate studies at Trinity College were interrupted when he joined the first Zionist Commission immediately after the First World War and spent a year in Palestine where he helped to found the *Palestine Weekly*. He was invited to join the London office of the Jewish National Fund where he became associated with the *Zionist Review*.

Returning to Dublin to take up his academic studies, he recognized immediately the remarkable talent of his fellow Dubliner James Joyce, of whose work he remarked, 'the riches are embarrassing'. Leventhal submitted a review of *Ulysses* to the *Dublin Magazine*; this was to mark the beginning of a literary association and deep personal friendship with its editor Seumas O'Sullivan, but as he corrected the galley sheets word came that the printers in Dollards would down tools rather than have part in the publication of the blasphemous writings of Joyce. In anger Leventhal wrote, 'A censoring God came out of the machine to allay the hell-fire fears of the compositors' sodality.' Determined that his review would appear in print, he produced a delightful magazine, *The Klaxon*, which introduced itself in strident tones:

We are the offspring of a gin and vermouth in a local public-house. We swore that we were young and could assert our youth with all its follies. We railed against the psychopedantic parlours of our elders and their maidenly consorts, hoping the while with an excess of Picabia and banter, a whiff of Dadaist Europe to kick Ireland into artistic wakefulness.

The Klaxon, lasting for only one issue (Winter 1923–4), was not permitted to achieve its nobly stated ambition, but it did at least publish a truncated version of Leventhal's article on *Ulysses*.

> In truth, there is no real parallel to Mr. Joyce in literature. He has that touch of individuality that puts genius on a peak. Rabelaisian, he hasn't the joie de vivre of the French priest; Sternesque, he is devoid of the personal touch of the Irish clergyman. Trained by the Jesuits, he can't guffaw like Balzac when he tells a good story. He is a scientist in his detachedness, but *Ulysses* is nevertheless, a human book filled with pity as with sexual instinct, and the latter in no greater proportion in the book than other fundamental human attributes.

After the demise of *The Klaxon* Leventhal became involved with another magazine *To-morrow*, which was to fare only slightly better than its predecessor in that it lasted for two issues, each of which had to be printed overseas to escape the moral rectitude of the Irish typesetters. It provided Yeats, Stuart, Lennox Robinson and Leventhal, among others, with a platform from which they voiced with an iconoclastic honesty their stifled sentiments on art: 'We proclaim that we can forgive the sinner, but abhor the atheist and that we count among atheists bad writers and Bishops of all denominations.'

Completion of a doctoral thesis was the signal for Leventhal's return to the academic world, and when Samuel Beckett resigned his lectureship in French literature at Trinity College, Leventhal was appointed to succeed him. The two became close friends, and of Beckett's many critics Leventhal is unique in his empathy with Beckett, a quality that gives to his comments on his friend's work an immense value. Leventhal saw in Beckett a genius even greater than that which had attracted him to Joyce: 'Beckett is in a sense a more intellectual writer than Joyce and his jousting with words has a background of erudition deeper, one suspects, than that of the master – the cher maître of the avant garde of the twenties and thirties in Montparnasse.'

It was Beckett's universality that elevated him, in Leventhal's view, above the mightiness of Joyce. Beckett was for all men of all time, even if 'Mr. Beckett's work is not for the many', whereas Joyce demanded for full appreciation certain preconditions: 'To appreciate Joyce fully one had not only to be a Catholic but have a Dublin background in addition ...' Beckett's refusal to conform, his desire and ability to lift literature from the abyss of convention, his audacity and courage in daring to go further than Joyce, all appealed to Leventhal. 'It may well be,' he wrote of *Fin de Partie* in 1957, 'that there is still a public that believes the age of experimentation is not over, that profundity however painful, is still preferable to vapid reiterations of tried and tiring formulae.' Above all, it was his friend's ability to establish landmarks in literature that most fascinated him. '*En Attendant Godot* belongs to no school, it will make one,' he wrote in 1954.

Leventhal's contributions to magazines and newspapers are many and varied. He was for most of his life closely associated with influential periodicals. At Trinity he was assistant editor of the University Magazine, *Hermathena*. He was also a regular broadcaster from Radio Éireann and the BBC. After his retirement from Trinity College, he lived in Paris where he continued to contribute to Irish newspapers, to the *International Herald Tribune* and to *The Financial Times*.

The influence of Judaism in life and art is a recurring theme in many of Leventhal's articles and in his poetry. His appreciation of lesser-known writers such as Amy Levy and Hannah Berman was a characteristic of his literary awareness.

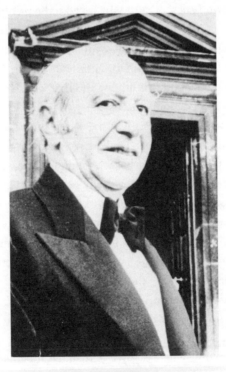

A.J. (Con) Leventhal.

Con was probably happiest in the theatre. Here the expressionism of literature could be projected in innovative form. For fifteen years he contributed a 'Dramatic Commentary' quarterly to the *Dublin Magazine*, and he has left a remarkable diary of Dublin theatre through the forties and fifties. The first of the series appeared in the October–December issue of the *Dublin Magazine* in 1943 and these continued until 1958. The strident tones, the felicitous style, and discerning criticism that were to characterize this unique diary of Dublin theatre during its fifteen years existence are evident in the opening lines of that first contribution in the forties:

> At its inception the Abbey Theatre incurred abuse to be followed by universal approval with a consequent acceptance at home like the prophet approved by proverb who only receives posthumous canonisation in his native town. Recognised in the first instance by the discerning few for the right reasons, praised by the equally discerning few in foreign parts, the latter brought their compatriots round to appreciation of a dramatic mode which despite a regional language and local dramatis personae, succeeded in crawling out of its provincial rompers to an adult metropolitan influence.

Leventhal's appreciation of theatre and the literature emanating from it, his affection for Irish drama and his empathy with actors and actresses (he was himself an accomplished performer) give to his criticism a warmth and feeling that is at the same time devoid of parochial sentiment. These qualities together with his familiarity with European theatre, and the all-embracing nature of Leventhal's interests make the 'Dramatic Commentaries' a valuable legacy in theatrical criticism.

The last contribution to the series was in the April–June issue of the *Dublin Magazine* of 1958, which also bears a poignant farewell tribute to the late editor Seumas O'Sullivan:

> As this Magazine goes to press we regret to have to announce the death of its founder and Editor, James Sullivan Starkey, otherwise Seumas O'Sullivan, the name by which he is known in the world of letters. From the first number of the *Dublin Magazine* in 1923 up to the present issue there is continuous evidence of the product of a mind with one standard – the highest. The list of contributors' names to be found elsewhere in this number, bears witness to Seumas O'Sullivan's catholicity of taste in poetry and prose. Many of these writers found their first platform in this Magazine. While Ireland's greatest writers shine magnificently in its files, there is no narrow nationalism. O'Sullivan could find room for English, French and American contributors if they fitted into his scheme of things. And through the annals of this journal there emerges the individuality of the Editor, stamping it with his brave decisions as much avant garde as traditional. Much will yet be written about

Seumas O'Sullivan as poet, essayist and editor, much about the man himself but there is little need to address the readers of this Magazine in this respect.

The future of this journal, now that its great artificer is gone, is uncertain. One would have liked at least one more issue in which writers could pay homage to this unique figure in the literary world. But many material and other considerations must be counted before a decision can be reached.

After his retirement from Trinity College, Con lived in Paris where he continued to contribute to Irish newspapers, to the *International Herald Tribune* and to *The Financial Times*.

Nevill Johnson

I FIRST MET Nevill Johnson in the early eighties when he was exhibiting at Tom Caldwell's gallery in Fitzwilliam Street. It was at this meeting that he gave me a copy of his autobiography, *The Other Side of Six*. Our friendship grew and when I published *The Beckett Country* in 1986, Nevill gave generously of his Dublin photographs, which were reproduced for the first time to a standard befitting their artistic merit.

Over the next two decades I visited Nevill regularly in his studio in Peel Street rescuing as many paintings as I could lest he paint over the canvases. These paintings and a number of Nevill's drawings were exhibited at the Solomon Gallery in Dublin in 1995. In 2002 I arranged an exhibition to mark the fiftieth anniversary of Nevill Johnson's photography of Dublin in the Lemonstreet Gallery, which was opened by Anthony Cronin. This exhibition presented for the first time a chronological account of Nevill Johnson's artistic career illustrated mainly through his photography, but also including his painting and writing. The photographs had their origin in 1952, when Nevill set out to portray the people and places of the 'real' Dublin of that time, revealing the privations and enduring strength of the inhabitants of the grand terraces, which had become slums, alongside the beauty and liveliness of the city. As an Englishman who had lived in Northern Ireland and Dublin since 1934 he was in the rare position of being able to endow his photography with the freshness of the outsider looking in while at the same time loving the city and its people.

I promised Nevill that I would see that his art was not forgotten and eventually took the first step to fulfilling this posthumous duty, when *Paint the Smell of Grass*, co-authored by the art historian, Dickon Hall and with an introduction by Nevill's son Galway, was published and launched at a retrospective exhibition in the Ava Gallery, County Down, on 25 November 2008.[8]

Paint the Smell of Grass, 1978

NEVILL JOHNSON was an enigmatic artist within whom three artistic *personas* struggled for expression. First, and dominant, was the painter in Johnson; then closely related but distinct, there was Johnson the photographer; and finally, Johnson the writer had to be content to let visual portrayal take precedence over literary expression. Serendipity cast him in four locations on the islands of Britain and Ireland. First, there was Buxton in the north of England, and the Isle of Man, where boyhood, family and schooling set down persuasive influences that would endure. 'Beneath the drawers, beneath the soft epidermal boundary of abdominal skin, not yet identified, named or recorded, lay a pulsing blastoderm. And there came to term in July 1911, under the sign of Leo, in one of the hottest summers on record, a blue-eyed web-toed left-handed boychild.'

Johnson's childhood and adolescence was dominated by middle-class comfort and privilege. His education was comprehensive and conservative, being directed to producing a predictable output to grace the academic or business establishment of pre-war England. But the system had a cuckoo in the nest.

> It is Armistice Day. I and my fellows are enjoying the unusual experience of being in the town. We line the main street behind a rope while there pass a succession of decorated floats to the sound of martial music. On one such float sits a shy Britannia, a local girl with helmet, shield and trident of wobbly cardboard. Our little band, dressed in Norfolk jackets and Eton collars wave Union jacks – all but me, that is. It seems that at the age of seven I already felt a need to stand aside, to walk against the wind.

Though art was not an influence in young Johnson's life there were at least two influences that would later become relevant. The King James Bible springs up in titles of many paintings – how much it was to influence content is debatable, but let us not confuse the enduring influence of this work of art with religiosity. Also from childhood were the pervading evocative influences of sight, sound and smell; indeed Johnson was to ask the same questions that had preoccupied Proust (and would later do so with Beckett):

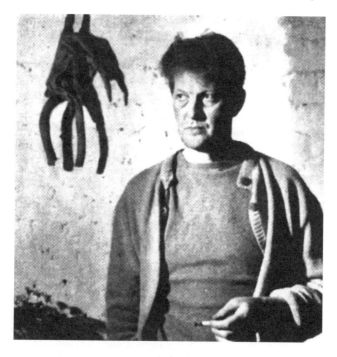

Nevill Johnson.

When you are nosehigh to a dog adults are but trowsers and skirts, so my parents and their friends were quite beyond my horizon. Right now my world was furnished with sunshine and warm stones, with close up grass and shoe-black beetles, and spiders on stilts. It was abundant with blackberries, and mushrooms budded like manna in the morning.

This artistic sense of evocation is further examined in a short passage from Johnson's autobiography *The Other Side of Six* in which he attempts to fathom the mind's remarkable ability to lock away a stimulus of evocation only to release it untarnished many decades later:

Presently I got to my feet and stood like a dog pointing. A certain smell, a perfume, attracted me, striking a deep memory; it was not the clover nor the meadowsweet, nor the camomile and the wild peas. I could not place it and, puzzled, returned to the sweet grass beside Sally trying to trace the memory. Way back I went – to a child of five leaning against the bank of a country lane in Anglesey in 1916. Some grass or flower on that bank released a perfume that profoundly affected me; part sweet, part fusty, like cloverhay or dried honeysuckle. For thirty six years I had remembered this smell with a tang of sensuality and melancholy, and had searched long to match this first rapture (for such it was), and on that August evening as the birds commenced to sing, as we brushed the seeds from our hair and made for the gate, I found it – in a tangle of flowers hanging from laurel – like leaves on the wall of the stableyard.

Johnson accepted the marvel of being that permitted the creative process but his thoughts were never too far removed from the scientific basis that facilitates execution of the wonder known as art.

It is said that the brain is a slightly alkaline electrochemical computer working on glucose at 35 watts. Be that as it may I stand always in awe of the depth and staggering range of man's memory, astonished by this bulging cornucopia – as I am daily surprised that, without heed or thought I stand upright, or wake in the morning. Thus, within the convolutions of my brain lie the sight and smell of unnumbered mornings, of seals sunning on the rocks and plover on the wind; of streams tumbling turfbrown from the flanks of Errigal; of Muckish glistening and Binyon, the lords and ladies of Donegal and Down.

When the time came for Johnson to conform, to become a member of the establishment for which he had been so well-groomed, it was not to be. He tried – but not for long:

One bleak morning I visited a hatter's shop and emerged in a few moments half shamed, half laughing wearing a bowler hat. Perhaps, thus covered, success would attend me? My father and brother wore them habitually. Let it be understood that I tried; it was just that my skull was the wrong shape for this adornment. I glanced up repeatedly to the driving mirror then pulled impulsively to the curb where I got out to the pavement and removed this expensive item from my head. I placed it upon the ground and crushed it with my foot. In this manner did I commit almamatricide.

Johnson fled to another part of the Empire – to Belfast in 1935, shedding in the process the comfort and security of family and business. 'There is a primitive within me, I think, that shies from the trap of comfort and complacency, which looks askance at rare carpets and the second car, which drips a little bile of discontent into our safe havens; a pattern-seeking logic-dodging ghost, refusing sanctuary and the easy option.' So it was to be – the future course had been charted.

But Belfast was a strange place in 1934: 'Institutional green and pew brown paint on those Presbyterian facades, few signs of style or culture. The trades basic; the making of rope and cloth, the building of ships. And rife here the Calvinist ethic. St Chads and Sedbergh had offered me no key to unlock the secret societies and their unspoken signals of complicity.'

Belfast was the beginning of Johnson's artistic career. Here he joined a circle of writers – Forrest Reid, Louis MacNeice and John Hewitt, and artists – John Luke and George MacCann. Luke influenced Johnson to take up painting for reasons that are not recorded, but what is evident is that once launched Johnson dedicated himself to painting with an intensity that only waned when periods of doubt obsessed him, as happened from time to time. Luke proved a good master and he had in Johnson a willing and talented pupil:

> It has not been revealed how this son of a shipyard worker came to be an artist and pupil of the Slade, nor do I recall how I first met this modest man. Suffice to say that he set about to teach me and set me spinning on my courses. For two years we worked together, patient John a good teacher. So, rising before dawn, painting early and late while earning my keep by day I worked without stint, fuelled by the distant hope of one day escaping from business.

The two travelled together to Paris where influences abounded:

> We stayed for a time in Paris exploring and tasting rare fruits. Braque and Picasso held sway and the surrealists were on stage; Ernst, Magritte and Tanguy, Lipschitz and Gargallo, splendid straight-faced progenitors of the furlined teacup and the spiked flatiron, tripping my pulse. And round the corner fresh young faces – Vivin, Peyronnet, Bombois, children of le Douanier, *maitre de la réalité*. Life enhancing stuff it was.

In Belfast Johnson met and married his first wife, Noelle Biehlman, a French-woman from Versailles, and had two sons. The couple escaped the oppressiveness of Belfast to the countryside to find peace and time to paint:

> So we moved to another farmhouse on the shores of Strangford Lough. Here was conceived our second son, and here I made for myself a private place reached by ladder in a little room over the cowshed. I was deep into Aquinas and Maritain – a peeping Thomist you might say. I flirted, to my astonishment, with Rome, taking instruction from the bland fathers; and was soon sickened by their responses to my modest though searching questions. I could feel no respect or tenderness for a Being so ineffably pure, beyond corruption. Compassion was stifled and I turned away, fancying myself insulted and demeaned by enraged angels. God knows what I sought but it was not to be found among the mystics and scholars of religious faith. I sought a saner world, far from patriotic fervour and a doglike 'smiling through'.

Religion was not the only demon to trouble the young artist. This was wartime and though Johnson would possess all the sensitivities to justify a stance as a conscientious objector, there was within him an inbred sense of loyalty and duty, instilled no doubt by an upbringing that was very traditionally 'old England'. Perhaps we should not be too surprised, therefore, to find the call to enlist for the motherland preying on his conscience.

> As darkness settled over the sea and the wind moaned in the chimney I sat thinking, suffering all manner of doubts and self questioning. Primitive defence of hearth and home I understood; I would rebut fascism from any quarter – but fight now for whom? For what? For King George, Mr Chamberlain, the 'B' Specials, the old school tie, the bums and bobbydazzlers? I was in a 'reserved' job, albeit that didn't resolve my problems and a few months later I entered a recruiting office on the Antrim Road – after a few drinks – and offered my life and services as aircrew. The offer was not taken up, but this did nothing to quell the voices within me – loyalty to what? To whom?

These doubts behind him, at least momentarily, the peeping Thomist firmly in its box, Johnson was free to make a declaration of independence from perfidy and humbug: 'Political and ecclesiastical societies were anathema to me; I disavowed all cults, clans and brotherhoods, as I avoided the hoods and headbags of cant, the polluted wine and the prejudicial bread. I thereby excited the attention of those devoted to surveillance, the notetakers and pigeonholers, the committed protectors of the status quo.'

The fishing village of Kilkeel on the coast of County Down was another retreat, a retreat that would provide the peaceful solitude needed to execute a number of paintings.

> The harbour rang with sweet sounds, on one side the thump and flash of an adze against the pale resinous ribs of a new built boat, its keel resting on grassy cobbles; and across the slow surging tide a band of men dressing granite, making curbstones for the streets of London. The unsynchronised ring of their chisels made water music, enhanced by the piping of sand martens nesting in the crumbling bluff which sheltered their simple forges from the wind.

But for Johnson, escape from a barbarous world in which man inflicted outrageous cruelty on fellowman was not possible, if for no other reason than the unimaginable suffering inflicted by one side was just as readily perpetrated by the other in the name of self-righteous retaliation and when viewed from the safety of a far-away pinnacle the overwhelming sentiment was a burden of unbearable guilt; a guilt, which if not to be expiated might at least be lightened through the sharing of pain on canvas. 'For myself and thousands more, these events demanded a total reassessment, a check time, a time to measure the burden of guilt, to reconsider the credit of being human.' Johnson has recorded these post-war sentiments in a brief chronology:

Diary of notable events 1945:

February 13th A cold night in Dresden, the citizens going about their evening business, washing dishes, bedding children. The Allies drop incendiary bombs and the city becomes enveloped in a firestorm, an inescapable holocaust, the streets like furnace tubes. Those people not burned choked to death through lack of oxygen. Total kill 135,000.

March 9th One hundred American bombers dropped firebombs on Tokyo, total kill 124,000.

May 8th End of European war. Body count 54,800,000 dead, 10,000,000 displaced.

July 2nd Japan sues for peace. Replying to a question by Mr Horabin in the House of Commons on December 5th – as reported by the *News Chronicle* – Mr Atlee said 'the decision to use the atomic weapon was taken at the beginning of July 1945'. The first atomic bomb was dropped on August 6th, and the offer of peace made by Japan was not accepted until August 10th.

August 4th Japan warned about the bomb.

August 6th Let us look closely at this summer day

I and my wife prepared a picnic for an afternoon on the shores of Lough Neagh.

John Luke scraped with a razor blade and polished with silk cloth a gesso panel, preparing to lay thereon an imprimatura or glaze of Ivory Black and Terre Verte.

The bones of Clegbert Chutz lay quiet in his grave in Morganza, Louisiana.

The ruins and the people of Hiroshima lay steaming and screaming in the evening sun. Colonel Paul Tebbitts, illustrating that strange paradox of submission to aggression enacted by all soldiers, had fulfilled his duty. Having centred his aircraft over the city he signalled release of the 9,000 lb bomb. It burst with the heat and blast of twenty thousand tons of TriNitro-Toluene above the living day – the scrubbing typing teaching eating nappychanging day. 97,000 people were blistered and destroyed, 10,000 died later of cancer and radiation sickness.

August 9th A second bomb named 'big boy' was dropped on Nagasaki.

It was inevitable that the South of Ireland would soon beckon as a haven from the turmoil of post-war Belfast, a broken marriage and the ever-present demon of doubt:

All artists are subject to periods of doubt, however, and I was no exception. It came suddenly; the painting was rubbish I felt, however well received; these silent surreal wastelands, these mute bones and raven skies – who was I addressing? Of what relevance are these Arcadian shores to a world of blackmail and bombs? In despair I ravaged the housekeeping pot and caught the train for Dublin. I had to see Victor, to have his assurance – though God knows he couldn't really help me. He provided lunch, brandy, money, warmth and flattery. I thanked him and left. But the brandy soon evaporated and the cigar became sour in my mouth. My song was a squeak I thought, my world a pretty place but gutless and unmanned. I was insulated, uncommitted – a touchline aesthete.

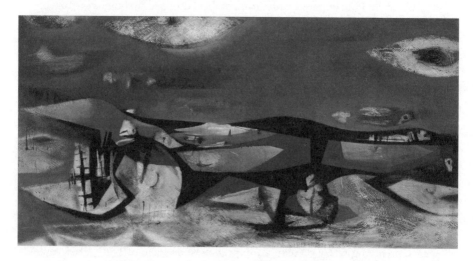

No Vile Men, *Nevill Johnson, 1956: oil on board, 12" x 16"*.

In Dublin, 'I closed one eye to make a friend – and found plenty.' Here his painting flourished. In 1946 Waddington encouraged Johnson to paint full time, offering him a retainer, and a regular allowance. He blended readily in the agreeable social milieu of the 'largest village in Europe'. The good dinners and cigars in Jammet's – courtesy of Victor Waddington – were relished, at least initially. This temporary security allowed Johnson time to reflect, to read more and to ponder his future. The work of Samuel Beckett is a constant refrain in Johnson's writings and he told me many years later that Beckett was an ever-present source of encouragement to him. We find a remarkable similarity in the artistic mission that each imposed upon themselves:

> Right now I lay on the bed smoking, thinking over the day's talk; of the creature who had enquired of me not only what sort of painting I made but why I painted. How answer that in words? Might as well measure distance with a thermometer – or pitch with a footrule. And that fellow reading Roland Barthes – who was this he quoted? Angelus Silesius (never heard of him). 'The eye by which I see God is the same eye by which he sees me' ... rum thought.

How similar these sentiments are to those of another artist – Samuel Beckett – struggling to find the meaning and the means of artistic expression.

Johnson's perception of Dublin in the fifties is important. He saw the city as one from without and unlike indigenous commentators, such as Cronin and Ryan, he had no need to eulogize the 'characters' of the city who, unlike those, such as Joyce and Beckett, with the guts to give the place the treatment it deserved by gazing back from afar, were being assiduously packaged and labelled for export to an outer world, which believed that leprechauns in green tweed strode the sidewalks of Grafton and O'Connell Street – and who would disillusion them? Johnson's view of Dublin did not deny the eccentricities of its people, the peculiarities of their behaviour, the hypocrisy of their beliefs, rather he saw the city for what it was and loved it all the more deeply: 'Through its people, thronged as they were by dogma and tacitly in thrall to the hereafter, ran a maverick undertow; these folk laughed and winked like boys behind Godmaster's back. Wit and a casual intelligence was the key to this society; today was fine – and tomorrow would be very welcome.' Johnson regarded Dublin of the fifties as a stimulating place and he may well have been right. It certainly bred an interesting array of talent provided the talent survived. 'The price was sometimes high; some drifted in a whirlpool of lost endeavour, some drowned … The bar stool supported some, others it captured, and for some the snugs were tombs.'

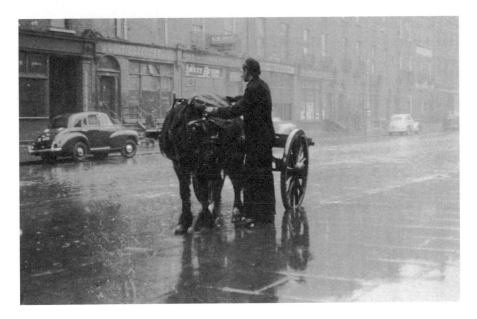

Pearse Street (Nevill Johnson).

The artist in Johnson sensed in Dublin what Dubliners themselves could not sense and what the planners of the next decade were oblivious to, namely that this capital microcosm had been suspended in time, its people as though from another age had been untainted by the evils of affluence that was contaminating the denizens of other capitals of the world; an aura of innocence and purity pervaded the place.

> Buttressed by piety, capped and shod by wit and crafty indolence, even the poorest lived out a strange Dickensian scenario. Behind elegant Georgian facades lay an intimate world of brick and iron, timber, and fine though crumbling plaster. The city had not yet undergone the humiliating submission to planners, and that frenetic consumerism which had begun to afflict the capitals of Europe. Day to day living passed unhurried, inexpensive, and a light-footed sanity prevailed.

The painter in Johnson set out to capture the uniqueness of Dublin but he substituted the lens of a camera for brush and canvas, and the result was a striking artistic success. Assisted by the artist Anne Yeats, Johnson walked Dublin of the fifties,

> circling like a hunting dog, nose and ear taking as much as my eye: the smell of hay and feeding stuff in a store off Smithfield, the yard paved with grassy flags and setts of old blue limestone. And there used to be a knackers' yard in Newmarket, whence came on west wind an evil stench of bones and hide.

In his introduction to the book he puts his case as a photographer: 'As Koestler says, quoting Paracelsus, "God can make an ass with three tails but not a triangle with four sides." So, in my photo-hat I cannot build or rub out – only select, and accept. I cannot in words translate the signals; I can only hope to match the image.'

Johnson's images of a Dublin lost are probably more valuable than any of the many notable photographic archives, such as Lawrence or Valentine, simply because in Johnson's case the photographer's eye is that of a painter; Johnson's images have a wonderful pathos because though intent on capturing a sense of place he did so by endowing place with its personalities, the residents, the joxers on the dole, the dockers, the clergy, the poor and down and outs, 'hosses' and bicycles, pubs and booze. Johnson's photographs of Dublin were not published for thirty years when, in 1981, a selection appeared in *Dublin: the People's City. The Photographs of Nevill Johnson 1952–53*, with an interesting introduction by Johnson and a foreword by James Plunkett. This publication was seriously flawed by poor reproduction that did a grave disservice to the photography. These unique images of a city and its people poised to step from an aeonian past into a turbulent future in which all would change utterly, must now surely be published in their totality in a sensitive format with duo-tone reproduction of the photography.

Another Dublin work of Johnson's that may interest the bold and daring is the *Symphonie Pour un Homme Seul*, later renamed *Goonstone*, a surrealistic cinematic romp in which love, violence, pornography and death are portrayed in Dublin, 'a total microcosm of a city on the life-supporting planet, Earth'. This work, which was never published, even less became a reality, is a film script filling some sixty pages of text. There are elaborate instructions as to how the complex series of flashbacks – present action in black and white, flashbacks in colour or sepia – are to be integrated. There was to be little dialogue because 'words have become suspect, devalued, hence *Goonstone*'s silence. He is not deaf – just wise.' The film is symphonic in form with seven movements and there are detailed directions for the sound sequences;

> The blackbird is used to denote tranquillity – and (in alarm) approaching violence. Apart from the Valse Grise accompanying smalzy sequences with Giggy, I want only natural sounds (Larks, corncrakes – becoming rarer through industrial farming), and man-made (peace-destroying) noises – Musak, M/C's etc. – except for Karl Orff's *Catullus* at the beginning of Adam and Giggy's love-making in Marram grass – which is followed by early Erotica.

Likewise the directions for character casting are clearly stated, for example, 'Anna – (Livia, Plurabelle, Molly/Ulysses) Earth woman. No ratting here. Sensual, quiet, content' and 'Giggy – sixteen on first flashback. Twenty-five on second flash-back. Kind, pinheaded, very sexy, passive, romantic blonde. A very sexy body.' As I said *Goonstone* is for the bold and daring but who will dare to fail?

In Dublin the painting went on – this was a prolific period for Johnson living in a variety of addresses – Raglan Road and Convent Place in the city and Ticknock in the mountains of Dublin. In the pubs the babble of witty conversation untainted by television or other distractions could be enjoyed:

> I stepped out to join a weird company; a throng of crazed polemicists, smart Alecs, winking know-alls, jokers and gentle men: In the pubs of Hartigan, McDaid, the Bailey and Byrne's, O'Dwyer, O'Neill and Mooney's on the bridge and after nighttime Powers and poteen, there were the characters – applecheeked O'Sullivan, Paddy Kavanagh, Augustan headed Behan and old Liam O'Flaherty, and 'Myles feeding our vanity and sanity in *The Irish Times*'.

Add to this the background figures, such as Harry Kernoff 'rising every morning from his bed into his hat', Denis Johnston, Mícheál MacLiammóir, and Con Leventhal, but to name a mere few and it is small wonder that one wag seeing Johnson approach his group exclaimed, 'O God, there are too many of us left.'

THE WEIGHT OF COMPASSION & OTHER ESSAYS

And women – always an important influence and necessity – helped sustain the painter: 'Amid these turbulent waters stood the bollards and mooring posts of my work. I had set up a teaching school, but my main income derived from wealthy ladies who desired to render the pretty colours of their gardens and drawing rooms; my "hollyhockers", I called them. A profitable exchange ensued.'

But even Dublin could not hold Johnson indefinitely. The city had served a need in him; he had served the city on canvas, celluloid and in prose. It was time to be off:

> I needed the wilderness – and a voice crying. In such mood I broke away from Waddington and jettisoned the bait; I brushed away the dust of Dublin and set off again for London – to be an exile in my birth land, to be an oddball in that country of class and compromise, that well swept catacomb of logic and commonsense. 'Why don't you give up painting and get a proper job,' they would say.

In Chalk Farm he was befriended by Cedra Castellain, who gave him a roof with fellow painters Robert Colquhoun and Robert MacBryde. This was a period when Johnson drifted, painting murals in clubs and bars. 'I took work where I could (*Dura Virum Nutrix*) as painter, decorator, any old job – creating nothing, but surviving, stoic, biding my time, a grailseeking misfit.' The lowest point came when he took a job as a milkman, leading his electric float through 'the cold dawns and misty streets' of London. 'I was rudderless though not yet beaten down.'

Then two happenings changed the course of his life. He met and married Margaret Pettigrew-King (alias Jenny in *The Other Side of Six*):

> Notwithstanding the requirements of legitimacy and the laws of property, I believed in divorce no more than I believed in marriage. The oaths and the written bonds, the witnessed registration of belonging, the receipts and waybills FOB, the licence to copulate – these were repugnant to me, an affront to the honesty of private declaration. We were married on a thundery afternoon at the registry office at Eye, Norfolk. Clad in torn jeans and jungle boots, I promised to cherish and protect, gaining thereby an oath of loyalty from Jenny.

He also inherited a little money with which he purchased four cottages at Wilby Green, near Framlingham. 'I had become a squireen, lord and master of fourteen rooms, four front doors and four privies.' Here he found solace and inspiration, in working the land and in communion with animals. He returned to painting: 'There followed a spring stunned with cold, and few birds left to greet it. Others perished that year: Georges Braque, Robert Frost, Jean Cocteau. I lived on, hoeing, digging, building – and now painting again.'

During this period Johnson kept a diary, which unlike *The Other Side of Six* is a very private chronicle without editing for publication, and, as such, is all the more valuable in permitting insight into the mind of the artist grappling with the artistic process, its joys and vicissitudes. The proximity of nature, the seasons however harsh betimes, the soil and animals, dominant themes in the diary, provide it would seem an ambience conducive to artistic expression, or at worst to contemplating how best to go about painting. 'Up at 7. The usual chore. Tea. Washingwater. Make the fire. Strong west wind, cool, good promise. Kitten shit everywhere. Biddy not well.' There was comfort and fun in the company of many friends who invaded the cottages at Wilby knowing that a kindred spirit lay inside: 'Constructed splendid cat walk for East window to by-pass painting table. Fully signed and directed.' It is interesting to see the artist instil into words the colours and the nuances of the canvas: 'Great skies. Thunder showers. Over-powering cumulus. Great snowy-breasted goose galleons of clouds. Greens and blues electric, the barley fear-pale.' Solitude was another boon though at times this weighed heavily: 'There is *too* much to enjoy alone. It is unbearable.'

At Wilby Johnson was able to indulge himself in reading and importantly to leave us some record as to what moved him in literature. He may have seen much of self in the disillusioned and exiled protagonist in Malcolm Lowry's 'compelling' novel *Under the Volcano*. He was also drawn to books on gardening, house building and magic, especially the 'fascinating' *Conjuror's Magazine* of 1793 with a translation of Johann Caspar Lavater's *Essays on Physiognomy Designed to Promote the Knowledge and the Love of Mankind*, which had so fascinated Goethe and William Blake among Lavater's many contemporary intellectuals. And in the background philosophers such as Henry David Thoreau emerge from time to time:

> A great cheerfulness have all great arts possessed, almost a profane levity to such as understood them not. But their religion had a broader basis in proportion, as it was prominent. The clergy are as diseased, in as much possessed with a devil as the reformers. They make their topic as offensive as the politician, for our religion is as impatient and incommunicable as our poctrial vein, and to be approved with as much love and tenderness!

Johnson was not much influenced by fellow artists but he did respect Robert MacBryde and Robert Colquhoun of whom he wrote: 'The local paper talks about McColquhoun the artist, now showing (God help him, with the advanced demographers of Museum Street). And Mr MacBryde. Don't mind Robert can still draw. I've seen them. Don't mind his company. OR his friends. And don't mind Picasso either.' Then on 21 March the diary records: 'Robert is dead. Collapsed & died in studio above museum gallery says East Anglian. Dear Jesus. Poor MacB. Poor everyone.' Johnson, never one given to expressing emotion, was deeply upset by this event: 'Rang S'OB from the Crown – it's true he's dead. More need to live. To use the time. O Jesus. I'm sad for him for him. This rare beautiful man. 47 for Gods sake. Idiot. Lovely man. Est is Bandt.' And later: 'I'm near to painting – nearer to Robert.' Other contemporaries in the art world get scant if not derogatory mention: 'Hockney (pop) shows at Kasmin. New Bond St Print Centre. Holland Street. W.8.' And Anne Yeats, who had trudged behind Nevill and his Leica in Dublin and who journeyed loyally to Wilby, receives the following: 'Anne Yeats entrained at Diss at 12.45. Nice, nice woman, but doglike. Mean of me, but so much to do – and so much treacle. Each way I even look, she looks. Like a mirror, and I'm not that pretty now.'

When I first met Nevill in the early eighties we found much common ground – life, beauty, women and, of course, the demon of the painting Byrne's Pub. In The Other Side of Six there is a delightful dissertation on alcohol: 'I examine the empty glass – fifteen pints a week by fifty-two weeks for fifty years: 39,000 pints. Yes. They should ring glad bells at opening time, I thought. O well, thus drank, no doubt Diogenes, thus Kepler, certainly Behan. Drinking is for younger men; provers, improvers, disprovers – and the hopeless ones.' A line from the Wilby diaries, 'Old jazz fetches me. I need dancing' brings back a fragment of our conversation at this first meeting, when Nevill told me that one of his favourite escapes was 'dancin' with nigga women in Camden Town'.

The last decade of Nevill's life was of necessity preoccupied with health, or rather lack of it. 'On shaky legs I entered the winter of my seventieth year, a sad bag of muscle and gut, humbled and prepared to listen. "Take it easy," they said, "and you'll last a few years yet."' He lasted quite a few years and painted away continuously and true to previous form destroyed much of his work. I visited him regularly during this period. One day as we sipped beer in the Churchill Arms, he invited me back to his little studio in Peel Street to 'share the mood he was transmitting to canvas'. I was astounded by the ten or so canvases he showed me. I asked if he had suffered much in their execution. He did not reply but asked why I thought there might have been pain. I felt in the paintings an intensity of personal involvement, an Augustinian expression on canvas.

He acknowledged that whereas the creation of a good painting might invoke great pain in the artist, the viewer might experience pleasure, no bad thing in itself, but a successful painting should also transmit the pain of the creative process to the voyeur, for such to a greater or lesser extent is the beholder. He then admitted to the constant presence of a 'monster' named 'doubt' that watched over his every brush stroke and made him wonder if anything he painted was worth a damn. Indeed, as I later recalled, he had identified the monster at a much earlier period in his career: 'All artists are subject to periods of doubt, however, and I was no exception. It came suddenly; the painting was rubbish I felt, however well received; these silent surreal wastelands, these mute bones and raven skies – who was I addressing? Of what relevance these Arcadian shores to a world of blackmail and bombs?'

Apart from the autobiographical catharsis that I saw in these paintings, I think I identified another quality I had seen also in Beckett's writing, and which I had earlier expressed:

> With this realisation comes another; much of the apparently surrealistic in Beckett's writing is linked, sometimes very positively, sometimes only tenu-ously, with the reality of existence, and much of this existence emanates from memories of Dublin, a world rendered almost unrecognisable by Beckett's technique of denuding his landscape and its people (while also annihilating time) in his creation of the 'unreality of the real'.

Was Johnson not expressing similar sentiments when he wrote,

> I spy psychiatrists and neurologists waiting in the wings. Let them come to the podium and state their case. Rupert Sheldrake, for instance, writes of time and spacedenying chreodes bearing atavistic messages from a deep primeval code through morphogenetic fields which determine our behaviour – and write our songs. Should I sit at this man's feet and thus quench the incandes-cent magic? I'm not denying the role of intellect; with it we can build a frame on which to pin our claims. Then, if the song rings true, we can kick away the props and it will stand.

The paintings from Johnson's last mood have achieved this; he has kicked the props to hell and the edifice is left resplendent in its sturdiness. The comparison that I have made with Beckett may indeed have more substance than we will ever know; as Beckett was influenced by painting, so too was Johnson influenced by literature not the least of which being Beckett's writings: 'In due course Samuel Beckett scraped the bucket of irony, while painter Bacon scored his canvas with torn flesh, and his screaming popes engendered a cult of intellectual ferocity and acting out the hopeless existentialism of the day, the day of Pozzo and the screaming cardinals of Bacon.'

I believe I restored Nevill's confidence that afternoon – at least for at time. I urged him to keep painting, not to compromise, to allow the 'mood of the moment' influence the brush. He needed though to escape from the stress of this 'mood' and we agreed that he would do this through drawing, which would allow him to free himself, to meander as it were with Picasso, Braque, the younger Johnson, or whomever. 'Such is the surge of delight that accompanies a good drawing; I am a privileged spectator firstfooting it in paradise – reopening for a moment that door which closed in childhood.'

On another visit to Peel Street, I realized that some of the paintings I had seen on my previous visit were gone and knowing that he only rarely sold a painting I asked him what had happened to *Golgotha*, which I had admired so much at our last meeting. He replied, 'Eoin, I devour my children.' I was put in mind of a line from *The Other Side of Six*: 'It is fair to say that I worked continuously at the painting – and destroyed all I made.' From then on my visits became missions of mercy with the purpose of saving as many of the 'children' as I could – some thirty or so – by taking them back to Dublin for framing for future exhibiting.

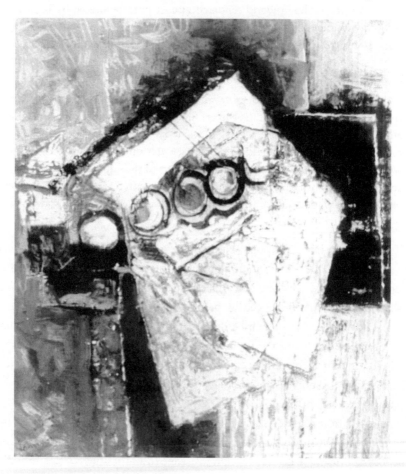

Golgotha, *Nevill Johnson, 1995: acrylic on board, 12" x 13"*.

During this period Nevill lived frugally; he had little income and he had not attempted to sell his paintings for years, and yet he saw his earlier works fetch, what seemed to him to be phenomenal sums. *The Family*, for example, sold at Adams Salesrooms in Dublin in 1991 for £20,000 and *Monkey, Harlequin and Women* for £9000. These and other salesroom successes rekindled interest in his work and one dealer made so bold as to suggest to him that he should paint again in 'the old style', recreating as it were the paintings of the forties and fifties, which were now proving so popular. This request enraged and depressed him and far from compromising his art for the babble of the market place, he determined to persist in the mood of the moment, which continued until his death. Two exhibitions of the 'children' of this last 'mood' ensued – the first at the Solomon Gallery in Dublin in 1995, and the second in the Tom Caldwell Gallery in Belfast in 1999.

On the literary front I was able to help Nevill complete his last literary work, the *Tractatus Pudicus*, best described perhaps as a poetic dialogue in which Johnson philosophizes on the human condition, and in the process gives interesting insights into his development as a painter. Take for example *The Hermit*, in which he expands on his friendship with his mentor John Luke (as originally recounted in *The Other Side of Six*), but he now expresses an opinion on Luke the artist (whose paintings are presently much sought after):

> Good day – can't stop. On my way
> to the shores of Arcady where dwell
> serendipitous P's and Q's.
> Where the still air bears witness
> and the buds envelop correct
> testimonials.
> All very welcome.
> It is time to tell a story. To tell
> it as it was.
> John Luke, artist, lived in a
> brick terrace house near the
> Belfast docks. His father lay
> in the front parlour a froth of
> spittle on his lips.
> Dead he was and waiting
> for the box.
> John had managed to reach the
> Slade where he sat at the feet
> of Mr. Tonks.
> He lived content

fine skinned
chopping twigs
defining his virginity
with gesso and yoke
of the unborn pecker
and Terre Verte
he built his sexless
Valhallas.

On my last meeting with Nevill some days before he died he looked from me standing at his bedside to the catheter draining him like an hour-glass that would alas never be inverted, and with eyes of sadness, sadness in the realization that his time had passed and mine not quite so, we parted on a quote from the Book of Samuel: 'How are the mighty fallen and the weapons of war perished.'

Denis Johnston

NIALL SHERIDAN introduced me to Denis Johnston and much more besides. I first met Niall at a dinner party in Eugene and Mai Lambert's house in the seventies. Niall was born in County Meath in 1912, where he witnessed the brutality of the Black and Tans in the family home, an experience that he never forgot and one that used to cause him considerable anguish in later life. He studied literature at University College, Dublin where he edited *Cothrom Féinne*, and numbered among his friends the literati of the day that included Denis Devlin, Brian Coffey, Arland Ussher, Denis Johnston, Michael Scott, Con Leventhal and Brian O'Nolan [Flann O'Brien, Myles na Gopaleen]. He is portrayed as Brinsley in O'Nolan's greatest book – *At Swim-Two-Birds*. The two visited Joyce in Paris in the thirties bringing Jameson whiskey and Haffners sausages, which greatly pleased Joyce and soothed the nerves of the two young authors. Niall served as a Senior Executive to Radio Telefís Éireann and in this capacity he arranged for me and Denis Johnston to accompany him one day to view his classic interviews with Denis and Sylvia Beech.

Niall was a marvellous raconteur with a prodigious memory and knowledge of literary and social Dublin in the middle third of the twentieth century. A glorious example of Niall's wit and mischievous humour is evident from our friendship with the musician Malcolm Arnold. Malcolm, who was born in Northampton in 1921, came to Dublin in the seventies to escape some domestic difficulties and

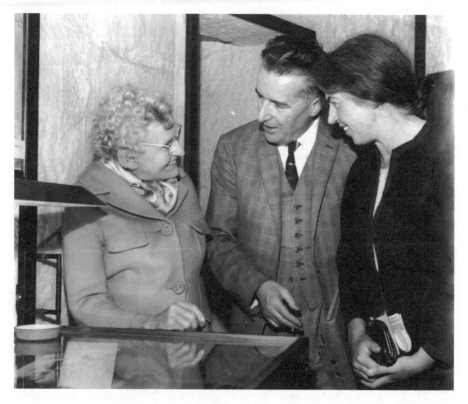

Sylvia Beach, Niall Sheridan and Mary Lavin at the Joyce Tower, 16 June 1962
(courtesy Niall Sheridan).

became enraptured with the city and its inhabitants. In particular he befriended Niall and Monica Sheridan. Malcolm had begun his musical career as a jazz trumpeter but soon devoted himself to composition writing nine symphonies and many concertos for contemporary musicians, among whom were Julian Bream, Julian Lloyd Webber, Benny Goodman and Larry Adler. He wrote the scores for many films including *The Bridge on the River Kwai* and *The Belles of St Trinian's*. Malcolm died in Norwich in September 2006.

During his time in Dublin, we met often and travelled to many restaurants – Malcolm's epicurean sensitivities were only a short step behind the demands of his music. However, on one occasion Malcolm developed some difficulty in passing urine and who better to perform the surgical niceties than a fellow musician who also happened to be deft with the scalpel. David Lane, who played the oboe and who served with me in the little hospital, known as Monkstown Hospital (alas now closed and demolished) was quick to recommend circumcision. This cured the ailment and the musician basked in the warm and tender care of the nurses in the hospital, where he received visitors with great delight and glasses of carefully chosen wine. Niall Sheridan deemed the occasion too great to be allowed to pass into oblivion without acknowledgment and wrote the following panegyric:

Now that the surgeon's work is finished,
Must Malcolm play a fifth diminished?
No! Mighty monarch of the trumpet,
Full many a tired but happy strumpet,
Awakening, blear-eyed in the morn,
Recalls that monumental horn.
Not Giscard, Kissinger nor Heath
Could such a noble sword unsheath,
And leave behind a relic – slight,
But subject to full copyright.

And so, dear friends, be not afraid
At hidden treasure now displayed;
No need to worry any further
When Priapus comes out of purdah;
No need to tremble or beware
The fate of Sampson minus hair.
Fear no diminuendo. Mark,
He's kept the trunk but shed the bark.
And with this happy thought I close;
It's no skin off the Master's nose!

This verse caused great merriment in Dublin and none was more pleased than Malcolm, who vowed to set it to music to be played with a brass band and full chorus in Cardiff Arms Park. Alas this composition (as far as I know) never became reality.

I tried on many occasions to persuade Niall to put pen to paper offering to provide secretarial assistance should it be needed, but alas Niall abhorred the discipline of writing, preferring the freedom of conversation, and we are the poorer for not having his reminiscences. I did manage, however, to persuade him to write an article for the *British Medical Journal* and assisted (hardly the word for one whose powers of recall were such that he virtually wrote the article without recourse to the quoted works) in what might be best termed an amanuensis capacity. This is one of the finest articles written on the subject of medicine and literature.[9]

I am grateful to Niall for bringing Denis Johnston and me together. We met often in the ensuing years, sometimes alone, sometimes with Niall and occasionally with Betty and Tona. Denis had had an interesting life. He was born in Dublin in 1901. He went to school in St Andrew's College and witnessed the Easter Rising from the proximity of the family home in Landsdowne Road. He studied Law at Christ's College, Cambridge, became a reporter with the BBC during the war and was awarded an OBE for his war reporting from North Africa, Yugoslavia and Buchenwald. His plays include *The Old Lady Says 'No'* (1929); *The Moon in the Yellow River* (1931); *The Bride for the Unicorn* (1933); *Storm Song* (1934); *The Golden Cuckoo* (1939); *The Dreaming Dust* (1940); *Strange Occurrence on Ireland's Eye* (1956); and *The Scythe and the Sunset* (1958). He published a biography, *In Search of Swift*, and two autobiographical volumes, *Nine Rivers from Jordan* (1953) and *The Brazen Horn* (1968 and 1976). Johnston's play *The Old Lady says No!* was originally submitted to Lady Gregory at the Abbey Theatre bearing the title *Shadowdance*, but it was returned by W.B. Yeats with 'The Old Lady Says "No!"' scrawled on it, so the author retitled it and sent it to the Gate, where it was first produced on 3 July 1929.

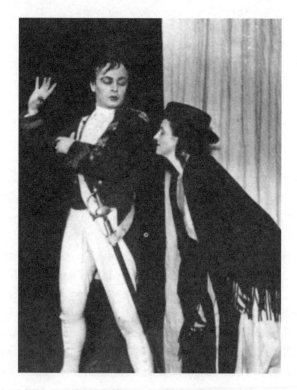

Mícheál MacLiammóir and Meriel Moore in the first production of The Old Lady Says No! *in 1929.*

My most poignant memory of Denis is the evening of 17 February 1977 when he asked me if I would accompany him and Mícheál MacLiammóir to the revival of *The Old Lady Says No!* in the Abbey Theatre. I collected Denis and we drove to the theatre where we met Mícheál and a friend and went straight to our seats. The play to be frank was quite bad and both Denis and Mícheál knew this. The only moment of light relief was when Emmet shouted, 'Is there a doctor in the house?' and Denis turned to me and said 'Now's your chance!' After the performance Denis preferred to remain in his seat rather than go to the bar. He was not in a talkative mood and I left him to himself, leafing through the programme without I suspect reading it too intently and when the audience had dispersed we left quietly. My overriding thought at the play and afterwards was one of sadness. I tried to fathom how both men must have felt almost a half-century after the first production, when by all accounts MacLiammóir in the role of The Speaker (Robert Emmet) was outstanding.

The following essay was first published in the *British Medical Journal* in 1978.[10]

Nine Rivers from Jordan, 1978

SOME TIME AGO I remarked to a friend that reading no longer gave me my usual pleasure. My appetite had gone; I nibbled everything, but savoured little; many books were started but few were finished – a literary climacteric, I reckoned. A few days later my faithful mentor presented me with a book, saying, 'This is what you need. Read it. You will find it interesting.' Thus did I discover *Nine Rivers from Jordan. The Chronicle of a Journey and a Search* by Denis Johnston. Having re-read the book – fearful on the one hand of shattering the magic of the first reading, but anxious to prove that its power was not illusory – I unhesitatingly rank *Nine Rivers from Jordan* as one of the most remarkable books of our time.

Denis Johnston is less well known than he deserves. Dublin, in characteristic fashion, is showing signs of belated appreciation, an occurrence that Mr Johnston may view with some scepticism. Born in 1900 and educated in Dublin and Edinburgh, Christ's College, Cambridge, and the Harvard Law School, he promptly abandoned the Bar for the theatre, having his first success in 1929 with *The Old Lady says 'No'*. (The title, incidentally, is a reference to Lady Gregory's refusal to stage the play at the Abbey and has nothing whatever to do with its content.) In 1931 *The Moon in the Yellow River* possibly his best theatrical work was produced at the Abbey. After this came many more plays and an iconoclastic work on Swift, which baffled and irritated the scholars. In 1942 he joined the BBC as a war correspondent, and *Nine Rivers from Jordan* is a chronicle of this period. He has called it a war autobiography, but it is very much more than that – it is the odyssey of a man in search of self and truth amid the chaos and horror, the humour and sorrow, of a global war. 'In the beginning is the Myth, and the Myth is Now and this Now is an illusion.'

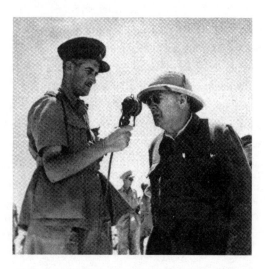

Denis Johnston interviewing Winston Churchill at
El Alamein (1943).

How readily we take for granted the technology of modern communication. It was very different in the early forties: cheating red tape and fellow correspondents to a scoop; cutting a disc in what seemed impossible circumstances, with relatively primitive and cumbersome equipment. Then the vagaries of transport to the ever-vigilant and ruthless censor before the final broadcast from London – this was the stuff of wartime communication. The truth, then as now, was just as illusory, and unacceptable: 'Our reporter, speaking from the Alamein Box quotes General Pienaar as stating that the line cannot possibly be held and that the Prime Minister in Washington is talking balls.' A German woman with a tender voice lulls two armies to sleep under a romantic desert sky with, 'Die Einst Lilli Marlene' – a poignant vignette? The censor does not think so: 'I thought you were supposed to be on our side.'

The frustrations of these early days were considerable, and at times there was the temptation to send a cryptic 'Upshove Job Arsewards' to London. 'All that I have to do is to give the world the facts. But the trouble is, there are no facts.' The facts are whatever one wants them to be, and at times it is necessary to create them

– Johnston's account of the Battle of Matratin was largely his own invention but, nonetheless, became the official version. The opportunity to do a first recording of a bombing raid gives Johnston the chance of a world scoop. The tedium, the terror, and the awesome beauty of the twelve-hour dummy run from Palestine to Benghazi makes the author seek solace in his paperback copy of Dante's *Inferno*:

> Over the desert in a stately shower
> Like snow upon the windless mountain
> Great flakes of fire are raining down.

Finally, there comes the great moment. The first-ever recording of a bombing raid (over the Tunisian seaport of Susse) becomes even more memorable for the remark, 'Here comes the F– shit', as the flak begins to come up. There are other scoops – interviews with Monty and the Old War Horse, but none greater than the perilous trip from Italy to interview the partisans on the transadriatic foothold of the Allies – the island of Vis.

Historical audio recordings are dispatched to London, including one of the Yugoslav partisans singing 'Tipperary' (in the mistaken belief that it was the British national anthem). From London come the compliments: '... they (the BBC) broke off the one o'clock bulletin for a special announcement ... Two BBC war correspondents had taken recording gear behind the German lines in Yugoslavia and made some outstanding recordings.' But, from an anxious Betty in Dublin comes an abusive letter enclosing a cutting from an English newspaper: 'BBC men risk lives for a song.' The greatest scoop lay farther into Yugoslavia. Johnston was offered an interview with Tito, and one suspects that he never forgave the authorities for not authorizing it, and himself for not ignoring the red tape.

Cheated by a few hours of being the first correspondent into Rome, there is consolation in the humour of Delia Murphy, the handsome wife of the Irish Minister, whose first realization that she had been liberated was when a resting soldier whom she presumed to be German said, 'Say, sister. Come and park your arse beside me.'

There is much humour in *Nine Rivers*. People in strange circumstances are often downrightly funny, and war is the strangest circumstance of all. There is, too, the sadness and loneliness of bewildered soldiers. There are the colourful characters; Frank Thornton-Bassett thundering on Christianity from the hills of Jordan: 'It's a doctrine taught by a bunch of wild men who came up from that valley there, in order to denounce both church and state, and to proclaim something that they called the Kingdom of God.' Perhaps the most colourful of all is Wynford Vaughan-Thomas, alias Young Bullivant, 'with a bright red face and a ridiculous beret, a dirty waterproof, and a wild zest for life dancing in his eyes'. A blasphemous pair, this Irishman and his Welsh *confrère*, dancing on the steps of the Basilica in Rome while singing 'The Old Orange Flute', 'for the delectation of the Roman populace' after the Pope's thanksgiving speech for the deliverance of Rome from war.

In spite of Johnston's regret that 'there are not enough women in this book … too many in my life, and too few on my arm', love and women glide through the pages. There is the loneliness of men separated from their loved ones (the homosexuals, at least in war, having the last laugh), the women of Paris, Rome, and vanquished Germany, Anneliese and the Pieta, and the hilarious fantasia at Madame Blanche's: 'The lovely little creature in the cage kicks up a dainty foot and a small silver slipper comes curling downwards through the scent-laden air. With blazing eyes I catch it, and filling it to the brim with the bubbling, icy Bollinger '28, I drink a toast to her loveliness in one long passionate draught.'

What matter if the reality is only myth? In the background there is a very real love story subtly narrated, in fact scarcely narrated at all, and all the better for this. Who is Betty, and why has he left her in Dublin? An odyssey in search of self we said earlier, a selfish odyssey as all such must be. Meanwhile, a divorce proceeds tortuously: 'If a few solicitors can make complete strangers out of two people who once loved each other, what chance in hell has an Englishman of understanding a German?' Johnston reports a world war in Europe, but what turmoil has he left at home? A brief interlude takes us to tranquil Dublin, to the poignant reunion with Betty in the Gaiety Theatre (where, as Desdemona, she is about to be murdered in her bed), and then to Belfast, by command of General Eisenhower, for marriage to his beloved.

What is it that guides our destinies? Is it the supernatural in the guise of a god, or are we at the mercy of the unpredictable winds of chance? How does a trivial event of today become the crucial influence of tomorrow? Or is it merely retrospective analysis that permits the irrelevancy to become the starting point of a revelation? In *Nine Rivers* certain occurrences lead inevitably, it seems, to the climax by way of a complex web of preordination: love letters from an unknown German soldier to his girlfriend Anneliese in the Thuringian village of Eckarts-berga are found in an abandoned German staff car in the desert; a dragoman reading Johnston's palm by moonlight at the base of the Great Pyramid presages the crossing of the nine rivers; his pact with himself not to carry arms in return for safe passage. These early events blur almost to insignificance in the advance on Mittel-Europa. But then suddenly he is in Ekartsberga, 'like some prophecy fulfilled, in spite of oneself', looking for Anneliese, but finding instead an American officer who directs him to Buchenwald and the truth at last, the horrible truth. 'Oh Christ, we are betrayed. I have done my best to keep sane but there is no answer to this, except bloody murder.'

> I went in. At one end lay a heap of smoking clothes among which a few ghouls picked and searched for what, God only knows … And as we came in, those with the strength to do so turned their heads and gazed at us; and from their lips came that thin, unearthly noise. Then I realised what it was. It was meant to be cheering. They were cheering the uniform that I wore.

He emerges a changed man, a man who up to this point believed that 'the jerry' was just another soldier doing his job. He had gone through the war without bearing malice to anyone (except possibly the censors), but now, blinded by this outrage to humanity, he violates his vow and pushes a souvenir – a Luger – into his pocket. Death is not too far off on the Brenner Pass. Was it to be a spiritual metamorphosis rather than a physical demise? 'When you know how to suffer, you will be able not to suffer. Who I am, you shall not know until I go.'

The post-war generation of readers may have difficulty in following Mr Johnston's peregrinations, but he does excuse himself: 'I feel a little guilty … in not trying to write history. Yet there are plenty of people who will do that, but not so many who will put on paper what it was really like.' Denis Johnston has succeeded in this ambition. Not only has he described war from an unusual vantage point; he has done so by bringing to his work the same innovative flair that made him a master of theatre. The prose is unconventional, occasionally a little uneven, but never dull. There are two intermezzos – an examination of conscience according to the Catechism and a 'critical exagamen' of his literary ability in which Joyce, Beckett, and O'Brien are parodied with effect and an old score with Yeats is settled. The Bible, the Tain, and Faust are introduced in ways that their authors would not have anticipated. Unfortunately the book is out of print at present, but it is available in most libraries. Aware to the dangers of adapting one form to another, I cannot, however, banish the notion, which perhaps more than any other describes my feelings on *Nine Rivers from Jordan* – it would make a bloody marvellous film.

Mícheál MacLiammóir

MÍCHEÁL MACLIAMMÓIR was born Alfred Willmore in the Kensal Green neighbourhood of London. He achieved acting fame as a child in the company of Noel Coward. Later when touring in Ireland he met Hilton Edwards and became captivated by the Irish language and culture, which he sought ways of adorning and elevating throughout his life. He co-funded the Gate Theatre, which thrives to this day. I first met MacLiammóir with my father, and I recall the whispered references to homosexuality, which to a schoolboy in Catholic Ireland simply did not exist and even later in student days was seen as something of a malady that could be wished away. I first saw MacLiammóir acting in two one-man shows of immense beauty and strength *The Importance of Being Oscar* in 1960 and *I Must be Talking to my Friends* in 1963. He painted and wrote many plays and books, one of the most enjoyable being *All For Hecuba*.

The essay on Mícheál follows a chance meeting with him on the ferry from Rosslare to Le Havre in July 1976, when he was accompanied by Paddy Bedford and Hilton Edwards en route for a tour of Provence.[II] Indeed seeing the trio I was reminded of a story that went the rounds of Dublin gossip some years earlier. Hilton and Mícheál were entertaining at their home in Harcourt Terrace. Answering a persistent bell Mícheál was greeted by Paddy Bedford, somewhat in his cups, with: 'Jasus Mícheál, the jacks, where's the effing jacks?' to which Mícheál replied, 'Proceed, my good man to the end of the hall where you will see a door with the sign Gentlemen, but let this not deter you for a moment and proceed straight in.'

On the Saint Patrick, 1978

Or what worse evil come
The death of friends, or death
Of every brilliant eye
That made a catch in the breath
W.B. Yeats

IN JULY 1976, aboard the *Saint Patrick* bound for Le Havre from Rosslare, I waited my turn in a long queue to a small hatch from which a sullen girl served a murky coffee. Suddenly, my spirits lifted on hearing an unmistakable rich voice proclaim, 'Hilton, do you mean to say that they are unable to separate the milk from the tea on this damnable tub?' And there, standing with a dripping paper cup held aloft, was Mícheál, looking bereft and very much out of place in this crowded eating hole. Placated eventually by Hilton, he sat alone at a small table smoking and gazing wistfully towards the sea. I introduced myself, and, although it was some years since we had last briefly met, he welcomed me warmly to his table.

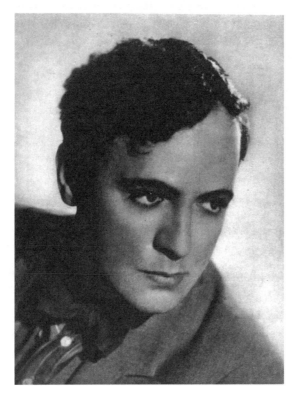

Mícheál MacLiammóir.

Of the *Saint Patrick* he understandably had little good to say. 'My dear boy, it is, I imagine, the closest one can come to a floating Belsen. It is unspeakable – one cannot travel like a gentleman any more. A young woman attempted to oust me from my cabin at nine o'clock, but I stuck fast – how awful.'

When I recalled meeting him in Harcourt Terrace when I was a boy, he expressed joy at my childhood remembrance. But he was, as he went on to explain, glad to have left home temporarily: 'You see, my partner and I have suffered so much there recently. Poor Hilton was in one room absolutely racked with pain. He has arthritis of the most painful variety and, furthermore, his obsession with the wretched television set resulted in excessive devotion to tennis, and he developed – to add to his other afflictions – tennis elbow while watching Wimbledon.' Warming to the topic of television, he went on:

> I must tell you a story. I was in a play, many years ago, in London. What it was I cannot remember. I was staying in a hotel at Lancaster Gate. Such was the design of the place that, on my way in and out, I had to traverse the lounge wherein nestled the television set. Every day, no matter what the hour, there sat in front of the set a young girl gazing at the machine with a look that could only be described as idolatrous. Eventually, after three weeks, I could stand it no longer. I marched up to her and said – 'My child, do you never go to the park to play with the other boys and girls?' She, without taking her eyes off the set, and barely opening her mouth replied in Cockney, 'Don't like boys and girls.' 'Well, my child, do you not ever take the dog for a walk?' 'Ate dogs, I do.' 'Dear, dear, don't you ever take the cat for a walk?' 'Simply 'ate cats completely, I do.' 'Dear, dear, my child, don't you ever read Hans Christian Andersen?' 'Oos ee?' 'He writes fairy tales, my child.' For the first time, she lifts her eyes from the television and looks at me as though I had come from another planet. 'O Gawd, don't be spoofy.'
>
> Well my boy, I said to myself, God help us if this is what we can expect from the future generation. And another thing television has done is to destroy manners. I was in the Yellow Rooms in Rathfarnham recently with an acquaintance, and, in passing a gentleman – we may at least call him that for the moment – who was standing at the bar with his pint clutched in his large hand, I unwittingly knocked his elbow and said: 'My good fellow, I am so sorry.' To which he replied, without moving, 'So you fucking well might be.' Lucky I was not to get my eye blackened, because he was quite a big fellow. Oh dear me, television has destroyed manners, utterly destroyed manners – how terrible.

I expressed my doubts about the effects of television on children, and this led Mícheál to his own childhood.

I attended what is known as a boarding school in England for one-and-a-half years, during which time I learnt endurance and the rudiments of arithmetic. I then went on the stage at the age of ten years, and was educated thereafter by my sister; who had a certificate for teaching. She used to teach me – I remember it so well – from a silky covered purple book. She took me from Chaucer to the Elizabethans, and, of course, to the greatest Elizabethan of all, and then through to contemporary authors – how I loved it. You see, my boy, keeping the hours that I did in the acting profession, regular education was out of the question. My father, of course, wanted me to take a business career – he later sent me to Spain to acquire Spanish for this pursuit, which I did.

'Happily, you did not pursue this vocation,' said I.
'Yes, happily for business.'
Continuing his childhood reminiscences, Mícheál went on,

I remember earning fifteen shillings a week when I started, and then, because I was good, I was given a leading part – it was, I think, in *The Goldfish Bowl* – and this brought in the large sum of £2 a week. My mother thought we were millionaires. But, dear me, I did not really know what I wanted to be, which was quite in contrast to another little ten-year-old who was playing with me – he knew exactly what he wanted to be, even at that age. 'An actor, Mícheál, an actor I shall be' – the cheek of the little pup, he was like that always even in later life, dear Noel Coward. Then I played in *Macbeth*. I was the apparition and Duncan's child. I had, of course, to be killed, and it was funny when as the apparition wearing a silken veil, and with my throat gashed, the veil caught fire at the cauldron and had to be quenched by the witches. Ha, Ha! Those were the times.

I declined a cigarette, pointing out with some regret that I had given them up.

Yes, you lose something, and I suppose you gain something. Smoking is a peculiar habit. It is not really a pleasure other than in a negative sense. Colette, that superb creature, put it so well; she said, smoking really minimises discomfort – if you are bored and smoke, you become a little less bored; if you are nervous and tense, you become a little less nervous and tense; if you are in pain, your pain is lessened. Don't you think that is the essence of smoking?

He went on to discuss Colette. 'Oh, how I would love to have met her. I adored her. She was, of course, old when she died in her eighties, I think. The world waited for Jean Cocteau, her great friend, to speak and satisfy its morbid curiosity about Colette. But, he was so shaken, so upset, and so honourable he was, as you know, queer, and she, the darling, was everything – that all he could say was:

"We loved as brother and sister, as man and woman, she was my dearest friend."
Don't you think that is beautiful, truly beautiful?'

A little later we reached Le Havre, and I waved goodbye to Mícheál and his travelling companions as they set off on their continental odyssey. I went on to Paris, haunted by a memory, his words ringing in my mind. No wonder he was so fascinated by Wilde – they were so alike in many ways. Unique artists with a common background – Dublin. May they enjoy pleasant converse in the Elysian Fields.

Petr Skrabanek

PETR SKRABANEK was a very dear friend, an exile from revolutionary Czecho-slovakia who made Ireland his home. We first came together in the Richmond Hospital where we shared an interest in neurology, probably because it is the most 'intellectual' of the medical specialities in that the diagnostic challenges posed demand an intimate knowledge of the intricate nervous system; furthermore, the diagnosis of neurological illnesses becomes truly akin to solving a complex cross-word puzzle, but then regrettably that is where the matter often ends without the neurologist being unable to offer much in the way of cure to his 'fascinating case' – the unfortunate patient, or such at least was the case when Petr and I toyed with being neurologists. We both later strayed to other reaches in medicine – he to epidemiology and the critical examination of medical dogma and me to cardiology.

We never lost contact for long and literature rather than medicine was our bond. This finally found expression in *The Cantos of Maldoror*, or more correctly failed to find that expression in that I have not yet fulfilled my promise to Petr to have his *limae labor et mora* published.

Born on 27 October 1940 in Náchod, Czechoslovakia, Petr studied chem-istry, entering Charles University in Prague in 1957. Following his studies he was a researcher at the Institute for Toxicology and Forensic Medicine in Prague gradu-ating in 1962. He then became the Head of the Toxicology Department in the

Institute for Forensic Medicine, Purkyně University in Brno. In 1963 he studied medicine at Purkyně University and in 1967 was selected to spend a month in Galway Regional Hospital where he met his future wife Vera in July 1968. This was the year of the Soviet invasion of his country and Petr found himself homeless. His love for Ireland was instant, destined to become a passion, a great affair in which our many weaknesses were seen in perspective against the beauty of the land, the personality of its people, their generosity, and perhaps above all their language both native and acquired. He came to the Aran Islands with no money, no prospects, and little English. Soon he had mastered Irish and the literature of the land to the extent of becoming an authority on *Finnegans Wake.* [12]

Petr was admitted to the Royal College of Surgeons in Ireland to finish his medical studies qualifying in 1970. For the next four years he worked in neurology in various Dublin hospitals. In 1975 he joined the Endocrine Oncology Research team in the Mater Hospital as a Senior Research Fellow and became involved in research into the neurotransmitter – substance P. In 1984, he joined the Department of Community Health in Trinity College with a grant from the Wellcome Foundation. Here he flourished bringing to the Irish a quality, which had once been theirs but which had been squandered at the turn of the century, namely the warmth and breadth of European culture. 'With the spirit of European iconoclasm he kept the medical evangelists in their hot boxes ... he chose to take the broader intellectual view of a profession in disarray, a profession in need of careful watching.' [13] Over the years he became renowned internationally for his outspoken views on many popular policies, especially when they sought to restrict people's freedom. The thrust of his philosophy, disseminated widely in papers and lectures, is to be found in *Follies and Fallacies,* which he wrote with James McCormick, and in *The Death of Humane Medicine.*

Honest expression soon draws detraction.

Shortly after his death Petr was accused of being in the pay of the tobacco industry – a 'paid stooge' to quote just one libellous vituperation – this from the *Guardian,* but, of course, the dead have no defence against slander. I examined the three 'tobacco-related pieces' to determine how Skrabanek earned his allegedly ill-gotten gains from the tobacco industry. In a letter entitled 'Smoking and coronary heart disease in women' Skrabanek cautions a *Lancet* editorial for having accepted without adequate epidemiological evidence an association in women who smoke less than fifteen cigarettes per day. In the letter 'Penalising smokers and drinkers' McCormick and Skrabanek take Sir Raymond Hoffenberg (then president of the Royal College of Physicians of London) to task for suggesting to a House of Commons Select Committee that smokers and alcoholics should contribute towards the cost of their treatment because their personal abuse placed a large financial burden on the NHS. The Dublin correspondents, alarmed at the pernicious implication of such reasoning coming from on high, if it was to be applied more broadly, for example to AIDS and intravenous drug abuse, reminded the president that tobacco tax alone raised annually a sum equal to one-third of total NHS expenditure.

'Smoking and statistical overkill' is a paper guaranteed to delight or irritate, depending on the reader's point of view, but in either case, it cannot fail to excite admiration for its incisive erudition laced characteristically with wit and humour. In it, Skrabanek attacks the use of alarmist tactics by doctors, epidemiologists, the media and politicians, who manipulate and pervert statistics to scare the public, which apart from being a tactic often based on falsehood, is one that has clearly been shown to be ineffective. By way of many examples, he cites WHO's dire admonition that half a billion of the world's population will be 'killed' by tobacco. All of which ignores another side to the equation, or as Skrabanek puts it 'even if everyone smoked, that would hardly put a dent in the world population, which is increasing by a million every four days'. Appealing against the use of large denominators to make a case, he asks that 'global' statistics be viewed through a 'global lens'. Warming to his task, he returns to that remarkable repository of statistical detail, the WHO: 'When a large denominator is used, even ordinary events make the head spin. For example, according to WHO over 100 million acts of sexual intercourse take place daily, resulting in 910,000 conceptions – 50 per cent planned and 25 per cent definitely unwanted – and in 356,000 cases of sexually transmitted diseases. Just in one day!' There is in this paper a passionate plea for the downtrodden of society (for me this is the foundation stone of Skrabanek's philosophy), the ill and infirm, the poor, the uneducated, the eccentric lost in the bottomless sea of epidemiological statistics. Can the epidemiologists tell us, he asks, how to advise a sixty-five year old widow, with rheumatoid arthritis, who smokes fifteen a day? 'For many people, whether soldiers, prisoners, loners, bereaved, the elderly, or the unloved, a cigarette may be the last friend and solace.'

He concludes with a plea for the human rights of the disadvantaged of society, those who are in danger of being isolated as 'pariahs' in the face of the seeming rectitude of 'responsible' citizens, who have the educational and general wherewithal to comply with the exhortations of the medical and political evangelists. 'Such polarisation can only speed up our descent into an intolerant, soulless, and dehumanised society.' Let us remember that Ireland offered Skrabanek sanctuary from just such a society. The Lancet's enquiry into the posthumous allegations upheld Skrabanek's 'stimulating and fearless stance on public-health questions', [14] and we can do no

better than harking back to the words of a former editor, Robin Fox, who extol-
ling Petr's contribution to medicine in 1996 anticipated perhaps the vituperations
that the future might hold, when he wrote, 'Gadflies should never expect a friendly
reception; Plato's associate Socrates suffered a more drastic form of peer review.'[15]

The translation of the *Cantos of Maldoror* is a tale of scholarship but added to
this is a delightful story of eccentricity in which a Dublin literary group set about
their task of translating Isidore Lucien Ducasse's masterpiece, not as might seem
fitting in the hallowed ambience of academe, but rather in a public house – The
Leopardstown Inn.[16] To plunge into the Maldororean seas is an experience that
can only enrich and the story around the Dublin *Maldoror* is one, like so many
Dublin epics, that draws on poignancy and humour – the tragicomedy of sorrow
and laughter.

The Cantos of Maldoror, 1997

LES CHANTS DE MALDOROR, written by Isidore Lucien Ducasse, otherwise
known as the Comte de Lautréamont, was first published in 1868. Petr Skrabanek
was first introduced to *Maldoror* around 1962 through the translation of Jaroslav
Zaorálek, sadly truncated due to the vigilance of the Czechoslovak censorship of
the 1920s. Bur Petr, being Petr, feeling the need 'to embrace my friend more inti-
mately', started to translate it for himself from the French. Aware that French and
English were not his native languages, he forged an intellectual alliance, first with
Dr Richard (Dick) Walsh, who taught phonetics at University College Dublin, and
later with Dr Gerald Victory, a devotee of Rimbaud (to whom he paid homage by
composing the ethereal *Cinq Chansons de Rimbaud*), francophone and Francophile,
polyglot and aesthete, with, in Petr's words 'an exquisite ear for the musicality of a
phrase'. All became infected by the strange beauty of the Maldororean sea.

This odd trio met in even stranger surroundings every Saturday at the stroke of
eleven AM in the Leopardstown Inn, a hostelry at the foot of the Dublin Mountains. Here week after week, year after year, every Saturday, they gathered with
their dictionaries, drafts, stacks of notes, pints of Guinness and glasses of Crested
Ten, all enveloped in clouds of tobacco smoke, blending with time into the decor,
so much so that the habitués scarcely cast them a glance. Then, sadly, to quote Petr,
'Dick decided to die.'

I came into the picture in 1992 when the translation was well under way.
Petr Skrabanek and I became acquainted as medical students but it was as young
doctors in the Richmond Hospital that we forged a friendship destined to deepen

and endure. I think it fair to say that we each admired something in the other that brought us above and beyond the intellectual restrictiveness of medicine. We indulged ourselves from time to time in whiskey, tobacco and above all conversation. I always departed such sessions enriched.

My first contact with Lautréamont was on a memorable evening in Dublin at a celebration in the Dublin Writers Museum to mark the publication of Samuel Beckett's first novel, *Dream of Fair to Middling Women*, in 1992 by Black Cat Press. Little did I know the saga that would follow that publication, but that is a Dublin story that must wait its time. What is pertinent to Lautréamont, is that after the formalities for *Dream* had been concluded, Petr tapped me on the shoulder, congratulated me and asked me if he could interest me in publishing a book on which he had been working for many years. In a corner of that elegant Georgian room on Parnell Square, he recounted the story of the Dublin *Maldoror*, concluding emphatically that it had to be published in Dublin, and he begged me to become involved as the text was not yet quite completed. Some weeks later I joined Petr and Gerry Victory at the Leopardstown Inn at eleven AM *sharp*. It was to be the first of many such sessions. Coffee was provided at regular intervals by the friendly curates until one PM, after which time alcohol was dispensed in various guises until we had spent ourselves on *Maldoror*, and each went his different ways until the next meeting. Such was to be the pattern until 1995. Apart from delighting in Ducasse's inventiveness and wonderful prose and agonizing over the nuances of a word, often for a whole session, we began to give more time discussing the ultimate publication of *The Cantos*. By this time I had scanned and entered Petr's typewritten text into the 'modern contraption' (as he liked to call computers).

Then a cruel destiny intervened. Sometime in 1994, walking along a corridor of Beaumont Hospital early one morning, I was surprised to see Petr coming towards me. 'What,' I asked, 'brings you to this establishment?' A look of profound sadness filled his eyes as he replied, 'Eoin, I am buggered, I have cancer of the prostate with secondaries in the spine.' We went down a quiet corridor an arm across each other's shoulder saying nothing and then I took him to the admission office. We now met more frequently but in Petr's home, where Vera served coffee and chocolate biscuits. Gerry and I watched our friend sink quite rapidly but he never relented on Lautréamont. My last memory of Petr is that of his wasted body almost smothered by the massive dictionary on his lap, the paroxysms of pain only quenched by the continuous infusion of analgesia, but Petr triumphant as the word that had eluded us all sprang from the dictionary and his smile derided the apparent hopelessness of his condition. Petr died peacefully on 21 June 1994 and went to join Dick and Lautréamont.

Gerry and I met on a few occasions with Vera to tie up some loose ends and then, as Petr would have said, Gerry decided to die on 14 March 1995. So Ireland lost one of its finest musicians and I wondered if Maldoror was not striding the plains of Erin and heading in my direction. But not being given to superstition, I soon returned to *The Cantos* and checked the numerous corrections that adorned many versions of the text.

The Dublin *Maldoror*, as I have called this translation, which sadly still awaits publication, joins four English translations of *Les Chants*. The first was John Rodker's *The Lay of Maldoror*, illustrated by Odilon Redon and printed privately in 1000 exemplars for the Casanova Society in Britain, in 1924. The next was an American version, *Maldoror*, by Guy Wernham, published in New York in 1943. The third translator, Alexis Lykiard, writes in the preface to his *Maldoror* (Allison & Busby, 1970) that Rodker's translation was 'an archaic travesty, full of elementary errors and misreadings' while Wernham's was 'even worse'. Lykiard's attempt is very readable, racy, and enthusiastic, but again with many errors. In 1978 *Maldoror* appeared in Penguin Classics, translated by Paul Knight. While being closest to the original, its language sounds stilted, words and phrases are left out and occasional misunderstandings of Lautréamont's twisted logic suggest that the work was done under time pressure. Even the title of the book, *Les Chants de Maldoror*, was not taken seriously by any of the translators, as they refused to translate *chants* as 'songs' or 'cantos', presumably trying to avoid the apparent conflict between the title and the prose of the book, thus missing the point of Lautréamont's mocking subversion of literary forms. Whether this humble attempt from Dublin to recreate *The Cantos* in English is any more successful is not for us to judge.

Two Russian Portraits

THAT TWO *fin-de-siècle* Russians should suddenly intrude on what until now has been a Dublin odyssey in literature and medicine is not as surprising as might first seem to be the case. Dr Chekov and Dr Korotkoff both shared a compelling sense of compassion that shaped their very different destinies. On first reading the proofs of my friend John Coope's revelatory book on Chekov, *Doctor Chekov: A Study in Literature and Medicine,* I saw that his achievements as a doctor and writer epitomized the 'weight of compassion'. There can hardly be a more poignant and courageous statement of the humanitarian sensitivity in the soul of the doctor than the journey of Anton Pavlovich Chekov to Sakhalin Island. To steal from a masterly article by Niall Sheridan, 'Here, surely, untouched by dogma, is a secular saint, the most attractive personality in the whole history of literature.' Here surely we have our epitome of the 'good doctor' but there is more to Chekov than his selfless dedication to improving the suffering of the underprivileged. He embraced literature in the scheme of being a good doctor: 'Medicine is my legal wife, literature my mistress.' This sentiment I believe is proof that these two disciplines – medicine and the humanities – can not only co-exist but that the one can enrich the other to the overall benefit of mankind.

And what of the other Russian doctor, Nicolai Korotkoff? Korotokoff, like Chekov, was driven by compassion for the poor and downtrodden in society, and like Chekov he died at an early age from tuberculosis. Korotkoff is remembered today for introducing in 1910 the method for measuring blood pressure, which continues to be used in medical practice. The history of blood pressure measurement is intriguing in itself but the man who first introduced the technique is the most fascinating part of the story.[7]

Anton Chekov, 1988[18]

'Medicine is my legal wife, literature my mistress.'

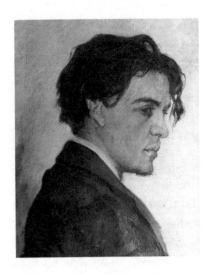

Anton Chekov.

TOLSTOY, a lifelong friend of Anton Pavlovich Chekov, said of his young colleague: 'Medicine stands in his way. He would be a much finer writer if he hadn't been a doctor.' Chekov would have disagreed; he never divorced medicine, his 'legal wife' – in fact, he remained faithful to her to the end – and she was a most demanding spouse. He also kept his mistress satisfied and she, likewise, was unrelenting in her demands. This remarkable symbiosis of Muse and Aesculapius is portrayed with delicacy and skill by John Coope in his fine study of Chekov.

Medicine gave Chekov the substance to fulfil the demands of his mistress. 'My medical studies have had a serious effect on my writing. They have taught me the art of how to classify my observations and they have enriched my observations.' Chekov like many other writers – Maugham, Carlos Williams, Gogarty, and Goldsmith to name a few – was also a doctor, but there the similarity should end. Chekov was unique among doctor-writers in being, first and foremost, an idealistic and hard-working doctor driven by his dedication to serve his patients, and whereas many doctor-writers continued to practice medicine, none I can think of did so in the sort of hell in which Chekov chose to immerse himself – the impoverished *zemostvo* system of rural Russia in which corruption, incompetence, and appalling deprivation were partners.

Throughout his life, Chekov never faltered in his belief in medical science. The disillusioned and depressed Andrei Yefimich, trapped in the hell of Ward No. 6, extols the advances that Chekov so admired:

> ... medicine has undergone a fantastic transformation in the last twenty-five years. In truth, what unexpected brilliance, what a revolution! Thanks to anti-septics, they perform operations the great Pirogov used to consider impos-sible, even in the future ... For a hundred abdominal operations, there is only one mortality, while gallstones are considered such a trifle that nothing is ever written about them.

In 1895 Chekov threw his energies into saving *The Surgical Chronicle*, one of Russia's few medical journals, and in so doing befriended medical editors of all time with the statement: 'A good surgery journal is as useful as performing twenty thousand operations.'

Chekov fought a personal battle with tuberculosis for twenty years, eventually succumbing to Koch's bacillus on 15 July 1904, at the early age of forty-four. Coope, himself a sensitive and caring doctor, who is familiar with the creative call, depicts perhaps as no other could, the pain and inevitable disillusionment that followed the first haemoptysis in 1884. We can at least be grateful that the infecting bacillus was not a virulent one, a fact that gave Chekov cause to doubt the diagnosis: 'If the haemorrhage I had in the district court had been the beginning of consumption I should have been in the other world a long time ago.'

Perhaps the most astounding aspect of Chekov's struggle with illness was his selfless disregard for his own welfare in pursuit of humanitarian causes. Not only did he dedicate much of his failing energies to founding (and financing) schools and hospitals for the peasants in Melikhova but he set out on an extraordinary odyssey to the convict island of Sakhalin. Coope brings new understanding to Chekov's determination to speak on behalf of the prisoners of Sakhalin, and of the punitive personal sacrifice this entailed. The hardships of this journey were truly frightful and he escaped death narrowly when his tarantass collided with three troikas, but it is the relentless misery and the sense of unremitting discomfort, not only on the journey, but also during his three-month sojourn on the prison island, that haunts the mind of the reader: 'We're driving on. The felt boots are as wet as a latrine. They squelch, and my socks are like a sopping wet handkerchief that you've just blown your nose in after a heavy cold. The coachman is silent and clicks his tongue despondently. He would gladly turn back but it's too late. Darkness is falling.'

Why, we ask, would a sick young doctor set out in primitive conditions to travel 5000 miles across some of the most inhospitable country in the world to uphold the cause of the detritus of society? The explanation may be found in a letter from Chekov to his friend A.S. Suvorin: 'I want to write one to two hundred pages and thereby pay off some of my debt to medicine, towards which, as you know, I have behaved just like a swine.' Would that such idealism might replace the avarice of contemporary medicine! And in the same letter, his thoughts on the pathetic plight of the unfortunate convicts on Sakhalin, afford us insight into Chekov's social conscience: 'All civilised Europe knows that it is not the warders who are to blame, but all of us, yet this is not a concern of ours, we are not interested.'

Chekov gained more at Sakhalin, perhaps, than even he could have anticipated – he saw into the very soul of the human condition, that which would later be enshrined in the Beckettian 'I can't go on, must go on.' The sadness and misery of Sakhalin, which so profoundly affected Chekov, cannot fail to leave the readers of this book untouched, even a century on, and so we are grateful when a benevolent destiny sees fit to bestow a little happiness on a weary physician returning from Sakhalin via Ceylon: 'When I have children I'll say to them, not without pride: "You fellows, in my time I made love to a dark-eyed Hindu maiden – where? – in a coconut grove on a starlit night."'

Back in Russia, Chekov wrote his expiation – *The Island of Sakhalin* – in which he drew the attention of Russian society to the plight of its convicts. This was not without effect, and in 1896 a government commission was sent to the island to investigate and make recommendations that helped to ameliorate the prisoners' pain and suffering that was to haunt Chekov for the rest of his days: 'I have rendered just tribute to learning and to that which the old writers used to call pedantry. And I rejoice because the rough garb of the convict will also be hanging in my wardrobe. Let it hang there.'

As an ardent admirer and student of Chekov, the writer, I am grateful to Coope for restoring to Chekov what I suspect is little known by even his most ardent literary followers, namely his dedication to the down-trodden – the unfortunate helpless of society. Indeed, had he lived in a later age, he would surely have earned a Nobel laureate for his persistent, masterly and sensitive exploration of this theme.

Nicolai Koroktoff, 1982[19]

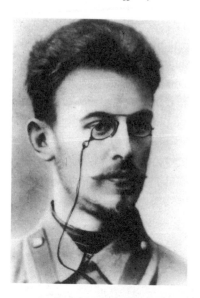

Dr Nicolai Korotkoff.

THE INFLUENCE of medical history on contemporary practitioners and on the course of medicine is as variable and subtle as it is contentious and ineluctable. Nonetheless, for most doctors there comes a time – especially in medical research – when they are drawn back to the pioneers of their specialty. Invariably they return enriched and refreshed from this temporal odyssey. How often one embarks on the journey in the belief that the terrain is unexplored, and how frequently this possessive zealousness gives way to mixed feelings of disappointment that so many others had travelled the same path, and relief that there is so much material to facilitate one's researches. There are, of course, exceptions but usually these are confined to the minor figures of medicine. Who would have thought that Korotkoff, a household name in clinical medicine, could have been neglected by medical historians? He is not even mentioned in Major's *Classic Descriptions of Disease*; Wilius and Keys ignore him in *Cardiac Classics*; and he fails to join the ranks of the great in Willius and Dry's *History of the Heart and Circulation*. Specialized books on blood pressure contain scant information on the man, although Lewis, Ruskin and Pickering attempted to redress the imbalance by publishing translations of his original paper from the Russian.

Nicolai Korotkoff has had, nonetheless, one staunch champion. Harold Segall took up the cause back in 1939, and a series of interesting papers have appeared over the years. The first published photograph of Korotkoff appeared only in 1970 and Segall produced another in 1976. These few papers provide us with the mere bones of biography; there is certainly no flesh, and hardly any sign of personality. Our own search for Korotkoff the man as well as the scientist brought us into a correspondence with Segall that provided tantalizing pieces of information with the promise of better to come. Then in August 1980 we received one of a privately printed issue of the first translation of Korotkoff's thesis and, of even greater delight to us, the edition included several unique photographs and a preface with biographical notes by Segall. The tortuous and prolonged research that makes this book so fascinating brings to mind *The Quest for Corvo*, with the difference that the quest for Korotkoff is not by any means complete. A review of the facts available may stimulate others – perhaps in Russia – to unearth more details about this enigmatic surgeon.

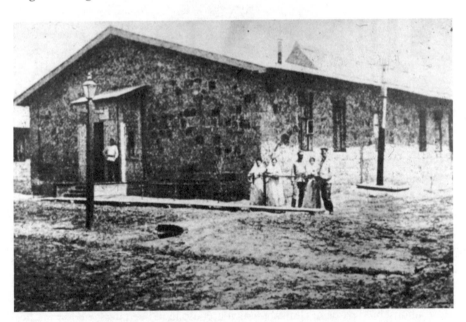

The building in which the second hospital of the St George Red Cross Society was lodged in August 1904 at Harbin, Manchuria (courtesy Harold Segal).

Nicolai Sergeivich Korotkoff was born to a merchant family of Orthodox faith at 40 Milenskaya (now Sovetskaya) Street in Kursk on 13 February 1874. He attended the Kursk Gymnasium (secondary school), where he received excellent marks for behaviour and diligence but was found wanting in 'divine law'. He entered the medical faculty of Kharkov University in 1893 and transferred to

Moscow University in 1895, where he graduated with distinction in 1898 at the age of twenty-four. He was appointed resident intern to Professor A.A. Bobrov at the surgical clinic of Moscow University. He is remembered as a tall, slender, studious young man, and his son recalls that his father attached great importance to the development of will power through self-discipline. On one occasion he almost took things too far when he plunged into the freezing waters of a river to test his determination, and became seriously ill from pneumonia.

Korotkoff was given leave of absence to serve with the Russian military forces in the Far East during the Boxer Rebellion in China in 1900. He was attached to the Red Cross in the Iversh Community under Dr Aleksinskii, a former pupil of Professor Babrov. The journey to the Far East entailed extensive travel by way of the Trans-Siberian railroad, through Irkutsk across Lake Baïkal to Vladivostock, and he returned to Moscow via Japan, Singapore, Ceylon, and the Suez Canal to reach the Black Sea and Foedosia. He was honoured with the Order of St Anna for 'outstandingly zealous labours in helping the sick and wounded soldiers'.

On his return Korotkoff turned his mind from military to academic pursuits and translated Albert's monograph *Die Chirtugische Diagnostik* from German to Russian. In 1903 Dr Serge P. Federov, an older colleague, was appointed professor of surgery at the Military Medical Academy at St Petersburg, and he invited Korotkoff to join him as assistant surgeon. In 1903 Korotkoff took the first of several examinations for a doctorate of medicine.

It was not long, however, before war again interrupted his studies. During the Russo-Japanese War in 1904–5, he went to Harbin in Manchuria as senior surgeon in charge of the Second St George's Unit of the Red Cross. He became interested in vascular surgery and began to collect cases for his doctoral thesis, which was to include forty-one reports of patients he had treated during his stay at Harbin.

Returning to St Petersburg in April 1905 he began to prepare his thesis, but it was a presentation to the Imperial Military Academy in 1905 that earned him lasting fame; the technique of blood pressure measurement was reported in less than a page of the *Reports of the Imperial Military Medical Academy* of St Petersburg.

> The cuff of Riva-Rocci is placed on the middle third of the upper arm; the pressure within the cuff is quickly raised up to complete cessation of circulation below the cuff. Then, letting the mercury of the manometer fall one listens to the artery just below the cuff with a children's stethoscope. At first no sounds are heard. With the falling of the mercury in the manometer down to a certain height, the first short tones appear; their appearance indicates the passage of part of the pulse wave under the cuff. It follows that the manometric figure at which the first tone appears corresponds to the maximal

pressure. With the further fall of the mercury in the manometer one hears the systolic compression murmurs, which pass again into tones (second). Finally, all sounds disappear. The time of the cessation of sounds indicates the free passage of the pulsewave; in other words, at the moment of the disappearance of the sounds the minimal blood pressure within the artery predominates over the pressure in the cuff. It follows that the manometric figures at this time correspond to the minimal blood pressure.

The critical comments of Korotkoff's peers were dealt with in an adroit manner, and he appeared a month later at the Imperial Military Academy with animal experiments to support his theory that the sounds he had described were produced locally rather than in the heart. He earned the approbation of Professor M.V. Yanovski, who declared, 'Korotkoff has noticed and intelligently utilised a phenomenon which many observers have overlooked.' These two brief communications are of greater interest to us than his thesis, which he successfully defended in 1910. Although he does refer to his technique of blood-pressure measurement in the thesis he does not describe it in any detail. In fact, were it not for Yanovski who saw the potential value in Korotkoff's technique, the auscultatory method of blood pressure measurement might have languished in obscurity. William Dock has taken this line of thought a little further, 'The most remarkable fact about the Korotkoff sound is that it was discovered.' Yanovski and his pupils verified the accuracy of the technique and described the phases of the auscultatory sounds. Yanovski was to Korotkoff as Samuel Wilks had been to Thomas Hodgkin, and for a time the technique was known as the Korotkoff Yanovski Method.

These three communications appear to be the sum of Korotkoff's contribution to scientific publications. In 1908 we find him serving as research physician to the mining district of Vitimsko-Olekminsky in Siberia. After receiving his doctorate he served as surgeon to the workers of the gold mines of Lensk. Here he witnessed some Tsarist atrocities, and was affected deeply by the murder of unarmed striking miners. After this he returned to St Petersburg and during the First World War he was surgeon to The Charitable House for Disabled Soldiers in Tsarskoe Selo. He welcomed the October Revolution, after which he was physician-in-chief of the Metchnikov Hospital in Leningrad until his death in 1920 at the young age of forty-six. His wife outlived him by twenty years and died in the siege of Leningrad in December 1941.

From these meagre facts some interesting questions arise. Firstly, did Korotkoff appreciate the importance of his discovery, and if he did was he not recalcitrant in failing to develop and apply the technique in clinical medicine? A study of Korotkoff's thesis shows that he had a keen intelligent mind with a researcher's appreciation of the value of a new technique, and even if we accept that initially he may not have appreciated fully the clinical application of his technique, he would certainly have become aware of it within the next decade as interest in blood pressure became international.

This brings us to the next question. Were circumstances, either personal or political, such that Korotkoff never had the opportunity to develop his discovery and indeed his scientific potential to the full? There are suggestions that this may have been so. He had shown, it would seem, sufficient academic promise to pursue a hospital career in St Petersburg or Moscow. He had translated Albert's monograph on diagnostic surgery two years after qualifying; he had presented his technique of blood pressure measurement aged thirty-one, and Fedorov had recognized his talent by inviting him to join his staff in 1903. What then prevented his academic development? It is possible that the criticism he received initially from his senior colleagues may have driven him from academe, but he appears to have been a match for his peers. Was it an interest in travel, or a desire to alleviate suffering, or merely circumstances that brought him to serve with the Red Cross units in the Boxer Rebellion in China and in the Russo-Japanese War in Manchuria? What was it that brought him to the mining district of Siberia, to the gold mines of Lensk, and to The Charitable House for Disabled Soldiers'?

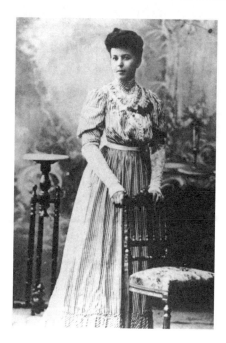

Mrs Nicolai Korotkoff (courtesy Harold Segal).

His wife also served in the Red Cross and accompanied him to Manchuria as a nurse. Perhaps we would not be wrong in scenting an aroma of kindly altruism in the Korotkoff household. This might account for Nicolai Korotkoff's apparent lack of interest in furthering his unique discovery. Indeed, it has been emphasized that one of the outstanding features of his personality was an intense 'modesty'. Perhaps this is not quite the right word, but to this characteristic has been attributed his rejection of an academic career and his refusal to develop, not to mind exploit, his scientific publications. Alternatively, his political beliefs possibly brought him into disfavour with the medical or political establishment. After all it is suggested that he left Lensk to return to St Petersburg after witnessing the murder of the striking miners. We are left wondering why.

Harold Segall in the course of his researches managed with the help of many friends to trace the son of Nicolai Korotkoff, Dr Serge Korotkoff, who specializes in 'sports medicine and rehabilitation with physical exercise'. It is heartening to learn that he is writing a biography of his famous father and an account of the evolution of the use of his father's technique (although, to the best of my knowledge, this has not been published). Dr Segall has happily undertaken to have the work translated into English, an event that will be an important landmark in the history of medicine. At the end of the day will Nicolai Korotkoff prove to be as fascinating as he is now enigmatic? It seems possible that he may.

George Frideric Handel

GEORGE FRIDERIC HANDEL'S unique gesture to Dublin and his support of worthy causes, not least being The Charitable Infirmary, was responsible for the production of *Messiah* in aid of medical research, organized by my late colleague and friend, John Fielding. The essay is reproduced from the programme.[20]

Messiah: An Oratorio, 1986

THIS PERFORMANCE of *Messiah* in the National Concert Hall, Dublin, on 2 February 1986 is an historic occasion for two reasons. First, it commemorates Handel's visit to Dublin, which gave rise to a musical event never surpassed in the city's long history, and his beneficence to The Charitable Infirmary and Mercer's Hospital. Of interest to future historians may be the uniqueness of the occasion, in that a commemorative performance to aid these institutes cannot be held again as Mercer's Hospital (already closed) and The Charitable Infirmary (shortly to be joined with St Laurence's Hospital) will not exist as the voluntary hospitals they were on the occasion of Handel's first performance of *Messiah* in the Musick Hall in Fishamble Street in 1742.

We may look back therefore from the vantage point of this historic performance to other events commemorating Handel in Dublin. A performance of

Handel's oratorio *Deborah* (composed in 1733) was held in 1748 to commemorate Handel's generosity to The Charitable Infirmary, and to raise funds for the hospital, when 351 tickets were issued to provide £194 10s 3d for investment. *Deborah* was performed annually in aid of The Charitable Infirmary until 1753.

In 1859, on the occasion of the Handel Centenary, *Messiah* was performed in Dublin in aid of Mercer's Hospital, and The Charitable Musical Society for the relief of distressed musicians. At this performance, Madame Goldschmidt (better known as Jenny Lind) was the major attraction.

In 1904 Handel's altruistic gesture to Mercer's Hospital was acknowledged on the cover of the *Mirus Bazaar* Programme on which his portrait and a piece of music from *Messiah* were featured. This bazaar at Ballsbridge was held in aid of Mercer's Hospital, an event that did not pass unnoticed by Leopold Bloom as he ambled up Molesworth Street to the National Library:

> Hello, placard. Mirus bazaar. His excellency the lord lieutenant. Sixteenth today it is. In aid of funds for Mercer's hospital. *The Messiah* was first given for that. Yes Handel. What about going out there. Ballsbridge

Later the viceregal equipage on its way through the city from the Viceregal Lodge in the Phoenix Park attracts the attention of Dublin's denizens, among whom is Blazes Boylan: 'By the provost's wall came jauntily Blazes Boylan, stepping in tan shoes and socks with skyblue clocks to the refrain My girl's a Yorkshire girl.' Boylan's generosity of spirit, if not directed towards the charitable needs of Mercer's Hospital, is at least, in communion with the festive mood of the city:

> Blazes Boylan presented to the leaders skyblue frontlets and high action a skyblue tie, a widebrimmed straw hat at a rakish angle and a suit of indigo serge. His hands in his jacket pockets forgot to salute but he offered to the three ladies the bold admiration of his eyes and the red flower between his lips.

In 1959 the Music Association of Ireland held a Handel Festival and Exhibition to commemorate the bicentenary year of Handel's death in the Civic Museum in Dublin.

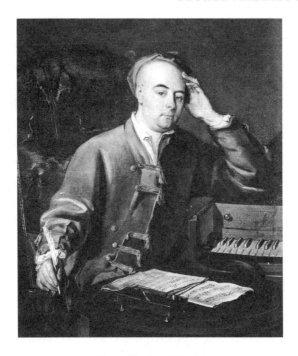

George Frideric Handel.

HANDEL IN DUBLIN

George Frideric Handel was born at Halle, in Saxony, in 1685 and died in London in 1759, aged seventy-four. A contemporary of Bach, with whom he shares a similar north German, middle-class and Protestant background, Handel was more flamboyant, gregarious and cosmopolitan than his compatriot. Described somewhat disparagingly by one critic as 'a magnificent opportunist', he composed nonetheless some brilliant music, of which *Messiah* is one of his finest achievements.

Beethoven regarded him as capable of achieving the greatest effect with the simplest of means, and Haydn in tears after hearing the 'Hallelujah Chorus' in Westminster Abbey, declared him 'the master of us all'. This sentiment would no doubt have pleased Handel, who had composed the chorus under the influence of great emotion: 'I did think I did see all Heaven before me, and the Great God himself!'

Handel was a profound Christian who gave generously of his artistic skill and reputation to raise substantial funds for charity. He was a governor of the Foundling Hospital in London to which he donated a magnificent organ. In the chapel of this hospital, Handel himself directed eleven performances of *Messiah*, so raising the sum of £7000 for that charitable institute. Handel's music was heard in Dublin probably as early as 1711, when the famous Italian castrato Nicolini sang excerpts (there is confusion as to whether or not the entire opera was performed) from Handel's *Rinaldo* in either the Smock Alley Theatre or the Blue Coat Hospital. In 1725 Signiora Stradiotti, the first Italian prima donna to grace the Dublin stage, sang a number of Handel arias at Smock Alley Theatre. On 1 May 1734 Handel's *Acis and Galatea* was performed for the first time in the Crow Street Music Hall. So Georgian Dublin music-goers were no strangers to the music of Frideric Handel.

On 2 October 1741 the new Musick-Hall in Fishamble Street opened under the management of Mr William Neale, one of a remarkable musical family who did much to further the appreciation and performance of music in the city. William Neale, a maker of musical instruments, was a member, with his father, of the Charitable and Musical Society, which organized musical events in aid of charitable institutes and causes. Subscription to the Society was an English crown. Meetings were held every Friday evening to perform a selection of instrumental music, after which the members entertained themselves singing glees and catch-songs. Concerts were given from time to time and the proceeds of each season were donated to a charitable cause, the most popular being the relief of debtors in prison.

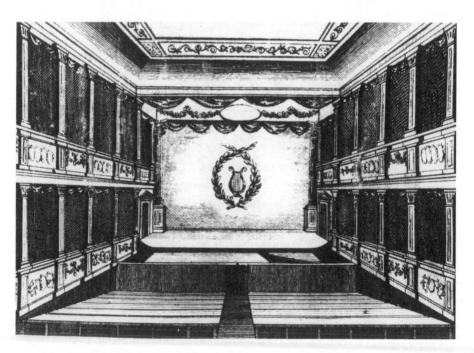

Interior of the Musick-Hall, Fishamble Street (courtesy National Gallery of Ireland).

The Society grew so much in popularity that it had to move from the Bear Tavern in Christ Church yard to the larger Bull's Head Inn in Fishamble Street. Taverns had never been in short supply on this little street and its history records the Swan Tavern, the Ormond Arms, the Ossory, the Fleece, and the London Tavern. The Bull's Head, which stood high on the west side of Fishamble Street next to St John's Church, was no ordinary tavern. Its extensive premises extended as far back as the east window of Christ Church Cathedral, and it has been described as 'a veritable ancient hostelry, with a capacious yard, which was entered by an archway, surmounted by the house's symbolic sign'. As a house of entertainment it had few equals. The Masonic Body had its home there, and it hosted the annual banquets of many guilds and public companies. Not everyone approved of the 'Bulls Head'; when Jonathan Swift, the Dean of St Patrick's, was informed that his vicars choral were members of the Charitable and Music Society, he called upon his subdeans to punish 'such vicars as should appear at the "Club of Fiddlers" in Fishamble Street as songsters, fiddlers, pipers, trumpeters, drummers, drum-majors, or in any

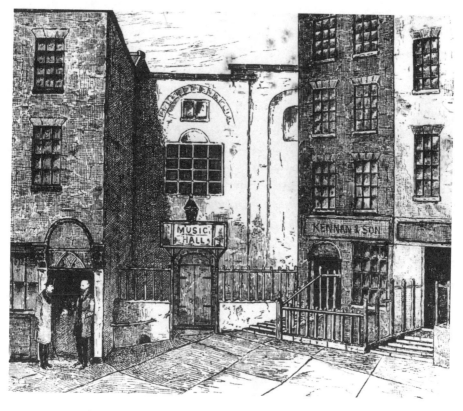

Exterior of the Musick-Hall, Fishamble Street.

tonal quality according to the flagitious aggravation of the respective disobedience, rebellion, perfidy, and ingratitude'. Despite such edicts the Society prospered, and funds were soon available to commission the building of the Musick-Hall to the design of the famous architect Richard Cassell, whom Bartholomew Mosse had brought to Dublin to build the Rotunda Hospital. The Musick-Hall when completed could accommodate seven hundred persons.

> As Amphion built of old the Theban wall,
> So Neal has built a sumptuous Musick Hall:
> The one, by pow'rful touches of his lute;
> The other, by the fiddle and the flute.

Fishamble Street, in the lee of Christ Church Cathedral, has an illustrious history. Once, as its name implies, a shambles or market for fish, the narrow way was lined with the open stalls of fishmongers, not always a cleanly lot. Their practice of casting the offal of their trade into the gutter in anticipation of the rains that would sweep it down the short hill to the Liffey was a source of constant irritation to the Corporation. The street once boasted fine examples of Dublin architecture, some of which dated from Queen Anne, including a number of tall narrow houses turning a high-peaked gable to the road. In one of these Henry Grattan, son of a physician, was born in 1746, and baptized in the Church of St John on Fishamble Street. Among other residents of note was Dr Arnold Boate, or Boot, brother of Gerald, the author of *Ireland's Natural History*, who, together with his brother, had written a refutation of Aristotle's philosophy. From the press of John Harding of Molesworth Court, off Fishamble Street, Swift's famous *Drapier's Letters* were issued in 1724. It is, perhaps, difficult to appreciate today the relevance of Fishamble Street to the history of the city, but it occupies no less than forty-five pages in Gilbert's *History of Dublin*!

With the foundation of Neale's Musick-Hall, the stage was set for the greatest musical event in the history of Dublin. Handel had become disillusioned with London society, where his concerts were being poorly attended. When the Duke of Devonshire invited him to visit Dublin, he was ready for a new venture and a change of air. Handel, always one to enjoy life, may have shared his biographer's opinion of Dublin as a city 'famous for the gaiety and splendour of its court, the opulence and spirit of its principal inhabitants, the valour of its military, and the genius of its learned men'. When the Lord-Lieutenant's invitation was followed by that of the Charitable and Musical Society, now proudly established in its new Musick-Hall, the maestro's mind was decided and he departed London for Dublin via Chester, where he was detained for nearly a fortnight by bad weather.

This delay may have been opportune. Having only composed *Messiah* a few weeks before his departure from London, Handel had had no opportunity to rehearse the music. This he did with the cathedral choir at Chester. The weather duly abated and Handel boarded the packet from Holyhead, arriving safely in Dublin on 18 November 1741. He took lodgings in Abbey Street, at which address tickets for his musical performances were sold. Handel's first concert in Dublin was announced to a public eager with anticipation:

> At the new Musick Hall in Fishamble Street, on Wednesday next, being the 23rd December, 1741, Mr Handel's musical entertainments will be opened, in which will be performed 'L' Allegro, il Penseroso ed il Moderato', with two concerts for several instruments and a concerto on the organ. To begin at 7 o'clock. Tickets for that night will be delivered to subscribers (by sending their subscription tickets) from 9 o'clock in the morning till 3 in the afternoon: and attendance will be given at Mr Handel's home in Abbey Street near Liffey Street from 9 o'clock in the morning till 3 in the afternoon, in order to receive the subscription money, at which time each subscriber will have a ticket delivered to him which entitles him to three tickets each night either for ladies or gentlemen.

The next entertainment was *Acis and Galatea*, on 20 January 1742. The programme also included an *Ode for St Cecilia's Day*, written by Dryden, and set to music by Handel. It was an astounding success: 'The Performance was superior to anything of the kind in the kingdom before; and our Nobility and Gentry, to shew their Taste for all kinds of Genius, expressed their great Satisfaction, and have already given all imaginable Encouragement to this grand Musick.'

The composer was also pleased, not only with his audience, but also with the acoustics of the new Musick-Hall:

> The nobility did me the honour to make amongst themselves a subscription for six Nights, which did fill a Room for six hundred Persons, so that I needed not sell one single ticket at the Door, and without Vanity the Performance was received with a general Approbation ... As for the Instruments, they are really excellent, Mr. Dubourgh being at the Head of them – and the Musick sounds delightfully in this charming Room, which puts me in such Spirits (and my health being so good) that I exert myself on my Organ with more than usual success ... I cannot sufficiently express the kind treatment I receive here; but the Politeness of this generous Nation cannot be unknown to you, so I let you judge of the satisfaction I enjoy, passing my time with Honour, Profit and Pleasure.

As with all great occasions, the organizers had their problems, one of which surprisingly, was traffic congestion:

To begin at 7 O'Clock, Gentlemen and Ladies are desired to order their Coaches and Chairs to come down Fishamble-Street, which will prevent a great deal of Inconveniencies that happen'd the Night before; and as there is a good Convenient Room hired as an Addition to a former Place for the Footmen, it is hoped the Ladies will order them to attend there till called for.

Acis and Galatea was followed by the dramatic oratorio *Esther*, which was received with similar rapture. Then, on 13 April 1742, *Messiah* was introduced to the world at the Musick-Hall in Fishamble Street, the proceeds to be donated 'for the relief of the prisoners in the several Gaols and for the support of Mercer's Hospital … and of The Charitable Infirmary'. The performance was, again, an outstanding success. The organizers of the Musick-Hall anticipating capacity crowds published a request that ladies would come without their hoops, and gentlemen without swords. The quaintness of this request should not be permitted to detract from its practical relevance to the occasion. The hooped petticoat had achieved its greatest dimension in the 1740s when it far surpassed 'both in circumference and stiffness the similar contrivance of Queen Bess's day', who had appeared to an irreverent wit as 'if she were standing up to her neck in a drum'. These considerations being complied with, some seven hundred people were accommodated in the hall for the performance, which raised the considerable sum of £400 for its stated charities.

The traditional observance of rising during the Hallelujah Chorus had to await the performance of *Messiah* in England, when the king rose to his feet. But at the Dublin performance, Dr Delany, friend of Dean Swift, was so overcome by Mrs Susanna Cibber's rendering of 'He was Desposed' that he struggled to his feet exclaiming on a note of emotion, no doubt soon to be regretted, 'Woman, for this, be all they sins forgiven.' The musical public of the city were enraptured: 'Words are wanting to express the exquisite Delight it afforded to the admiring crowded Audience; the Sublime, the Grand, and the Tender, adapted to transport and charm, the ravished Heart and Ear.'

Handel's last performance in Dublin was *Saul*, on 25 May, which was reported as 'the finest Performance that hath been heard in the kingdom'. During his stay in Dublin, Handel had visited the dying Jonathan Swift, who in his demented state had difficulty in understanding to whom he was being introduced, but at length exclaimed, 'O! A German, and Genius! A Prodigy! Admit him!'

Handel left Dublin on 13 August 1742 with fond memories of a city to which he resolved to soon return. Sadly for Dublin, and perhaps for music, this ambition of Handel's was never fulfilled. The musical public of the city did not forget the composer or his music, and the Musick-Hall, which continued to thrive long after Handel's departure, included his compositions regularly in its repertoire. The celebrated oratorio, *Judas Maccabaeus*, was performed there for the first time in 1748. William Neale, the successful manager of the Musick-Hall, had the satisfaction of seeing his son, John, become an accomplished violinist. He played often in his father's hall as a member of the Musical Academy, founded in 1757, by Lord Mornington (father of the future Duke of Wellington), for the relief of distressed families. John Neale had another interest, which in those bygone Georgian days was, to say the least, at variance with the sensitivities of a violinist; he was surgeon to The Charitable Infirmary, one of the institutions to benefit from the performances of Handel's *Messiah* under the auspices of his father's altruistic society.

Let us hope then, this evening, that Handel's spirit rejoices in hearing *Messiah* performed consummately again for the two institutes he so generously endowed. By our presence here in the National Concert Hall in Dublin, we not only support Handel's charities, but, in our appreciation of his music, we pay homage to the composer of one of the finest oratorios ever written.

Dominic Corrigan

MY FIRST INTRODUCTION to doctors who could contribute to medicine while also acknowledging the world of literature, antiquity and art was from my father, who loved music and poetry, and who regaled me in my medical studentship with stories of that brief moment in Irish medical history when the Dublin School was an international phenomenon in the Victorian world. From him I learned of Stokes, Corrigan and Graves, among others, who gave Dublin a place in the sun. But it was not until I was a registrar in training in cardiology at the Manchester Royal Infirmary that I began to seriously study the history of Irish medicine, and from this period I later published a series of essays, *Masters of Clinical Expression*, which included essays on the founders of the Dublin School – John Cheyne, Robert Adams, Dominic Corrigan, William Stokes and Robert Graves.

This initiation in medical history led to a long involvement with the medical and historical past of the city of Dublin, where I was to spend so many years in practice as a cardiologist. Ultimately, these influences found expression in *Conscience and Conflict: a Biography of Sir Dominic Corrigan 1802–1880*,[21] which was published to honour the centenary of Corrigan's death in 1980. It draws on papers, letters, diaries and memorabilia that had been left to the Royal College of Physicians and is a detailed treatise on his life and times.

As I embarked on my assessment of Corrigan's life I did so with a heavy heart. If one read the biographical note on Corrigan in the *Dictionary of National*

Biography, written by a London physician Norman Moore, it is likely that the urge to search further into Corrigan's life would have been quenched promptly. He denied Corrigan any priority in describing the disease and pulse that bear his name. This is the very best he can say on his behalf: 'His paper shows that he had made some careful observations, but he cannot have made many.' Even Corrigan's success as a practising doctor can, in Moore's view, be explained without having to bestow any personal credit:

> He had received little general education, and had no knowledge of the writings of his predecessors, but he was the first prominent physician of the race and religion of the majority in Ireland, and the populace were pleased with his success and spread his fame through the country, so that no physician in Ireland had before received so many fees as he did.

There can be few biographical notes in the *Dictionary of National Biography* that attempt to destroy so utterly their subject.

And yet a discerning reader should not fail to notice the extreme sentiments and sectarian undertones that in effect speak more of the writer's character than of Corrigan. However much one might have wished to examine the veracity of Moore's opinions, it would not have been easy to do so. Corrigan had faded into the mists of time without exciting more than a few laudatory obituaries, and a handful of essays that relied more on anecdote than fact. I remembered that the former librarian of the Royal College of Physicians, Gladys Gardner, had once mentioned some papers on Corrigan, possibly bequeathed by the family. I sought the help of her successor, Robert Mills. We found a trunk of Corrigan's personal and business letters, notebooks, diaries, pamphlets and memorabilia given to the College by one of his descendants, the late Francis Cyril Martin, in 1944, where they had remained undisturbed until the centenary year of his death.

These documents convinced me that there was a great deal more to Corrigan than anyone in this generation, and possibly in his own, realized. It was intriguing to discover how, coming from an artisan Catholic background, he rose from being a dispensary doctor in fever-stricken Dublin in 1828 to attain an appointment to The Charitable Infirmary where he achieved international eminence in medicine, and then went on to become president of the Royal College of Physicians of Ireland, physician-in-ordinary to Queen Victoria, a baronet of the Empire, a commissioner for national education, a senator of the Queen's University, and a Liberal member of parliament for the City of Dublin. The following essay is based on the 'The Dublin School' from *Conscience and Conflict*.

The Dublin School, 1983

IRELAND HOLDS a position of esteem in the annals of nineteenth-century medical history for the remarkable contributions to clinical medicine emanating from a movement that came to be known simply as the Dublin School. This title, correct in denoting the origins of the school and its role in the reformation in clinical medicine, does not, however, convey the dynamic idealism and iconoclasm that gave to this renaissance international recognition and the approbation of posterity. The School has been decked with many garlands, not least being the romantic title 'the golden age of Irish medicine', a tribute not undeserved, for at no time previously, nor at any time since, has Dublin had so great an influence in medicine:

Three 'giants' stand out from a galaxy of lesser, though by no means insignificant, luminaries who created the School – Robert Graves, Dominic Corrigan and William Stokes. If we seek qualities common to these three Irishmen, we may discern two outstanding talents: a compelling desire to observe the pattern and effect of illness with impartiality, even when their studies refuted conventional practice, and the ability to describe their observations with elegance and authority. Their courage in assailing the doctrines of established medicine was sustained by a clarity of vision cultivated in no small measure by their frequent travels abroad; they insisted on maintaining and fostering contact with their continental and American colleagues, realizing clearly as they did so that if Irish medicine was deprived of exposure to an active intellectual environment it would sink to mediocrity and flounder.

Indeed, it was the complacency arising from insularity, together with a dearth of talent to replace the founders of the School, which brought about its ultimate dissolution on Corrigan's death in 1880.

The personalities of the founders may fade into the shadows of time, but their contributions to medicine have been immortalized by eponyms with which medical students across the globe are familiar: 'Graves' disease', 'Cheyne-Stokes respirations', 'Stokes-Adams' attacks', 'Corrigan's disease', and 'Corrigan's pulse'. To appreciate the achievement of the Dublin School we need to look back to the Georgian doctors who laid the foundations on which these Victorians could build their temple to Aesculapius, and to examine the state of medicine in Ireland in the mid-nineteenth century.

THE GEORGIAN ERA

The standards of medicine in Georgian Ireland were deplorable, both in practice and within the organizations responsible for the regulation of the profession. The overall impression of the period must be, that with a few magnificent exceptions, the Georgian doctors of Dublin concentrated mostly on their own welfare, and did little to advance the practice of medicine. Such of course was the mood of a selfish age.

Following the suppression of monasteries in 1541, the monastic and religious houses throughout the country were closed. The closure of the Hospital of St John the Baptist in Dublin left the city without a hospital for nearly two centuries. Dr Richard Steevens, a wealthy physician, died in 1710 and bequeathed monies for the foundation of a hospital for the relief and maintenance of curable poor persons. To his memory must be credited the first successful attempt to found a voluntary hospital. He entrusted the execution of his will to his twin sister Griselda, who diligently applied herself to the task of building the hospital that now bears her brother's name, although its opening post-dated that of The Charitable Infirmary by fifteen years. In 1718 six surgeons determined to provide for the medical needs of the sick-poor, and The Charitable Infirmary was opened in Cook Street. This was followed by Dr Steevens' Hospital in 1733, Mercer's Hospital in 1734, the Hospital for Incurables in 1744, the Rotunda Lying-In Hospital in 1745, the Meath Hospital in 1753, St Patrick's Hospital in 1757, the Cork Street Fever Hospital and House of Recovery in 1804, Sir Patrick Dun's Hospital in 1818, and the Coombe Lying-In Hospital in 1823. In 1729 the notorious Foundling Hospital was opened by the government, and in 1773 the House of Industry Hospitals were founded from which developed the Hardwicke Fever Hospital (1803), the Richmond Surgical Hospital (1810) and the Whitworth Medical Hospital (1818). The background story to each of these hospitals is one of individual and corporate endeavour. The most remarkable philanthropic doctor of the Georgian period was Bartholomew Mosse, who by personal denial, selfless dedication, and a vision both classical and practical, raised sufficient money to build the Rotunda Hospital, a memorial to the architectural beauty of the age, which continues today to care for the lying-in women of the city.

Jonathan Swift, Dean of St Patrick's Cathedral, believed that the city of Dublin had a need every bit as compelling, if somewhat at variance to that which had motivated Mosse:

He gave the little wealth he had
To build a house for fools and mad;
And showed by one Satiric touch
No nation wanted it so much.

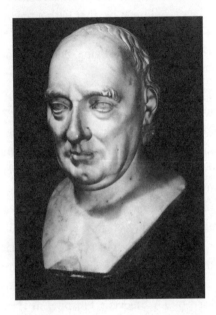

*Dean Jonathan Swift. Bust by Patrick
Cunningham (courtesy St Patrick's Hospital).*

John Cheyne, first professor of medicine in the Royal College of Surgeons (1813–19), was not Irish, but such has been his association with Dublin that his Scottish origins are often overlooked. John Cheyne would not be of great interest to us were it not for the fact that in 1846 William Stokes, in describing a peculiar form of respiration commonly found in terminal illness, recalled an earlier description by Cheyne and the condition is now known as 'Cheyne-Stokes respiration'.

The most illustrious member of the new College of Surgeons, and one who could, at least in terms of eponymous recognition, be counted part of the Dublin School, was Abraham Colles. Born in Millmount in Kilkenny in 1773, he graduated like so many of his contemporaries at Edinburgh. Colles returned to Dr Steevens' Hospital in 1799. Though his publications are fewer than those of his later contemporaries, the quality and content are exceptional. 'Colles's fracture' was described in 1814, and in his work *Venereal Disease* he challenged the well-established Hunterian view that secondary syphilis was not contagious, by stating what was once known as Colles's law:

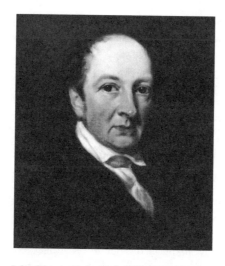

John Cheyne. Portrait by Rev. William Deey
in the Royal College of Physicians of Ireland.

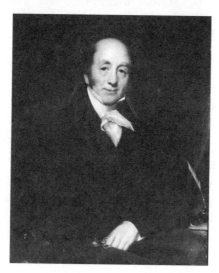

Abraham Colles. Portrait by Martin Cregan
in the Royal College of Surgeons in Ireland.

One fact well-deserving our attention is this; that a child born of a mother without any obvious venereal symptoms, and which without being exposed to any infection subsequent to its birth, shows the disease within a few weeks old; this child will infect the most healthy nurse whether she suckle it or merely handle it; and yet this child is never known to infect its own mother, even though she suckle it while it has venereal ulcers of the lips and tongue.

What Colles did not realize was that the mother had previously been infected, but nonetheless his deductions were for the time prescient. Dr Steevens' Hospital had a reputation for the treatment of venereal disease. In the 'fluxing' or 'salivating' wards patients were given under special nursing care courses of mercury, which is highly poisonous if given in excess.

Colles was a skilled surgeon but surgery in these early days before anaesthesia and antisepsis was, to say the least, primitive and often terrifying. In one of his papers there is a vivid description of an operation in which he attempts to tie off one of the main arteries in the chest to cure an aneurysm or swelling of the artery:

> And now it was found that the aneurismal tumour had extended so close to the trunk of the carotid as to leave it uncertain whether any portion of the subclavian artery was free from the disease ... the majority (of assistants) appeared disposed to abandon the operation altogether. Prior to tightening the noose (around the artery) the breathing of the patient had become more laboured and he complained of much oppression of his heart ... his countenance grew pale and indicative of instant dissolution ... some of the assistants were so strongly impressed with the idea of his danger that they quitted the room lest he should expire before their eyes.

Such hopeless efforts at heroic surgery were not uncommon and the outcome was almost invariably fatal.

Colles was a magnificent teacher, and in his lectures he attempted to inspire integrity as well as knowledge in his students: 'Be assured that in this, more than in any other walk of life, public benefit and private advantage are so blended together that the most certain means of advancing your private interest is to promote the public good.' He was devoid of political ambition and in 1839 he declined a baronetcy. In 1841, anticipating his death, he requested his friend Robert Harrison to have his body examined 'carefully and early ... to ascertain by examination the exact seat and nature of my last disease'. When he died, William Stokes in accordance with his last wishes, published *Observations on the Case of the Late Abraham Colles* in which the cause of death was attributed to a weakened and dilated heart, chronic bronchitis and emphysema of the lungs, as well as congestion of the liver, all occurring under the influence of a gouty constitution.

It is difficult, indeed almost impossible, for us today to appreciate the barbarism of surgery and the paucity of medical remedies in the nineteenth century. Many accounts of surgery in contemporary journals bear testimony to the cruelty of the operations attempted without anaesthesia, but none convey the hopelessness as vividly as the drawing by a student who was present at an operation for the removal of a malignant tumour from the left breast and armpit of one named

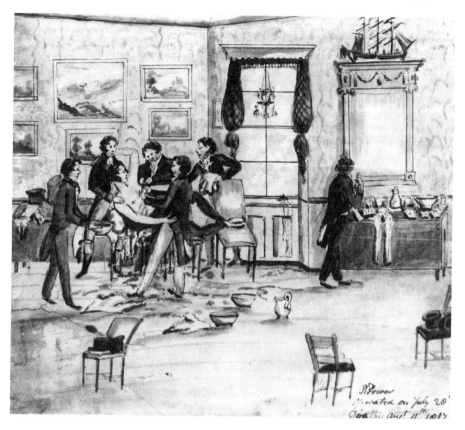

An operation in a Dublin drawing-room, painted by a medical student in 1817.

Richard Power in a Dublin drawing room on 20 July 1817. The surgeon performing the operation is Rawdon Macnamara (president of the Royal College of Surgeons in 1813), who was at the time only two years qualified and most probably apprenticed to Sir Philip Crampton, depicted in the coat and hunting boots. Even if patients survived the pain and calamity associated with major surgery, infection almost certainly claimed the victim, as it did the unfortunate Power within days.

If such was the state of surgery, the practice of medicine was little better. The actions of such drugs as were available were poorly understood, and most therapeutic remedies were directed towards counteracting the effects of inflammation, both general and local. With fever and suppuration accounting for the great majority of illnesses, the antiphlogistic methods of treatment had an almost universal application. These remedies consisted of bleeding, purging and starvation, and were often combined with techniques of counter-irritation, such as blistering, and the application of heat and cold.

The oldest of these techniques was blood-letting, which has been practised in one form or another by almost all cultures and societies. One method employed was phlebotomy or venesection whereby a vein was opened with a lancet or fleam, the blood then being collected in a bowl; alternative techniques were the local removal of blood by means of scarification, cupping, or the use of leeches. Large quantities of blood can be removed from a vein and the practice was often carried to extremes, causing the death of the patient. This was hardly surprising if the advice to 'bleed to syncope' was taken literally, or if credence was placed in the dictate 'as long as blood-letting is required, it can be born; and as long as it can be born, it is required'. The rationale of the technique was based on the fallacious belief that by turning the circulation of the blood from the centre of the body to the surface, the patient's-illness would be dissipated. The physician's reputation depended not only on his dexterity and grace in employing the lancet, but also on his judgment in determining the amount of blood to remove.

Of all the skills employed by the physician, that of cupping called for the greatest show of dexterity and professional aplomb. Cupping is one of the oldest medical procedures, and one that is not yet extinct even in Britain.

The technique is performed by heating a glass cup to exhaust it of air, and then placing the cup on the skin that is sucked into the mouth of the glass. After about ten minutes the capillaries in the skin burst, giving a painless bruise. This procedure is called dry-cupping, which may, if indicated, be supplemented by wet-cupping whereby the bruised area is scarified by several incisions (made with a special scarificator containing several small blades), and the cups are then reapplied to draw off blood. One glass could extract as much as four ounces of blood and it was common practice to place four or six cups on the back or abdomen, though most areas of the body capable of supporting a glass were cupped by practitioners of this art. Other antiphlogistic measures consisted of blistering, purging with laxatives or emetics sometimes given to maintain a state of continuous nausea, and finally starvation.

The drugs available were few and their actions poorly understood. Digoxin, morphine and quinine, which are still in clinical use, were available in the nineteenth century, but so also were strychnine and mercury, and there is evidence that all were used to excess. Doctors had not yet considered the concept of assessing the efficacy of treatment by controlled studies.

THE GOLDEN AGE

It was from this state of medical practice that the Dublin School was to arise. Is it possible for us from this distance in time to detect its origins? The international reputation of the Dublin School can fairly be stated to have had its very foundations in Robert Graves. He was born in Dublin in 1796 to a family whose forebears had come to Ireland with the Cromwellian army. Having spent some time at Edinburgh, Graves graduated from Trinity in 1818 at the age of twenty-two, and promptly set off to study at the famous European centres of Berlin, Göttingen, Vienna, Copenhagen, Paris and in Italy. His travels were not without interest and excitement. A facility for foreign languages landed him in an Austrian prison for ten days on the suspicion of being a German spy.

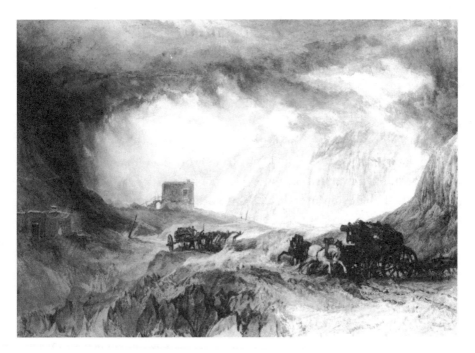

Passage of Mont Cenis, *J.M.W. Turner, 1819*
(courtesy the Birmingham Museums and Art Gallery).

While travelling through the Mont Cenis pass in the Alps in the autumn of 1819 he met a young artist and the pair travelled together for some time, neither seeking the other's name. Graves and his companion, whom he described as looking like 'the mate of a trading vessel', had a common interest – sketching;

together they painted and sketched as they travelled through Turin, Milan, Florence, and Rome. 'I used to work away,' Graves later recalled to Stokes, 'for an hour or more, and put down as well as I could every object in the scene before me, copying form and colour, perhaps as faithfully as possible in the time. When our work was done, and we compared drawings; the difference was strange. I assure you there was not a single stroke in Turner's drawing that I could see like nature; not a line nor an object, and yet my work was worthless in comparison with his. The whole glory of the scene was there.'

Graves was appointed physician to the Meath Hospital in 1821 at the age of twenty-five. His opening lecture did little to endear him to his seniors. He claimed that many fatalities resulted from indifferent treatment, and he deplored the attitude of medical students who walked the wards in pursuit of entertainment rather than medical knowledge. Graves had been impressed by the method of bedside clinical teaching on the Continent, especially in Germany. He praised the gentleness and humanity of the German physicians, who, unlike their Irish and English colleagues, did not have 'one language for the rich, and one for the poor' and whose practice it was to put unpleasant diagnoses into the Latin, rather than upset their unfortunate patients. Graves introduced the concept of notes to chart a patient's progress.

He was determined to reform the teaching system then practised in Dublin and Edinburgh, whereby students could qualify without ever examining a patient. Clinical teaching was often little more than an interrogation of the patient by the physician, with the results of the interchange delivered in poor Latin by a clerk to a crowd of students, most of whom could not even see the patient.

> The impassable gulf which in that aristocratic era lay between the student and
> his so-called teacher, was by Graves made to disappear and for the first time
> in these countries was the pupil brought into a full and friendly contact with
> a mind so richly stored that it might be taken as an exponent of the actual
> state of medicine at all time.

Together Graves and Stokes taught Auenbrugger's method of percussion, and both were experts with the stethoscope. They encouraged the student to take a history directly from the patient, then to examine the patient, to make notes and finally to discuss the diagnosis, pathology and treatment. Graves never forgot the patient: 'Often have I regretted that, under the present system, experience is only to be acquired at the considerable expense of human life ... The victims selected for this sacrifice at the shrine of experience generally belong to the poorer classes of society.'

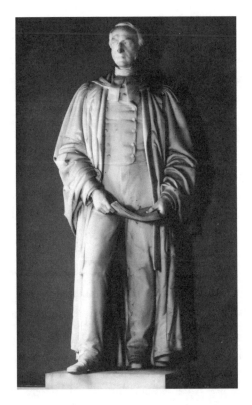

*Robert Graves. Statue by Albert Bruce-Joy in
the Royal College of Physicians in Ireland (D. Davison).*

In 1843 Graves published his famous *Clinical Lectures on the Practice of Medicine*, which was subsequently translated into French, German and Italian. In this book we find evidence of the gift that was common to these Victorian masters of clinical expression – the ability to describe their observations in clear and lively prose. Hale-White put it rather nicely: 'The lectures are unlike a modern textbook in that they can be read with enjoyment in front of the fire.' The famous French physician Armand Trousseau regarded Graves's book as a masterpiece:

> For many years I have spoken well of Graves in my clinical lectures. I recommend the perusal of his work; I entreat those of my pupils who understand English to consider it as their breviary; I say and repeat that of all the practical works published in our time, I am acquainted with none more useful, more intellectual.

In his preface to the French edition he wrote, 'I have become inspired with it in my teaching … when he (Graves) inculcated the necessity of giving nourishment in long continued pyrexia, the Dublin physician single-handed assailed an opinion that appeared to be justified by the practice of ages.' Here he was referring to Graves's revolutionary treatment of patients with fever, in whom he advocated supportive therapy rather than starvation, bleeding and blistering. The story goes that one day on his rounds, he was struck by the healthy appearance of a patient recently recovered from severe typhus fever and said to his students: 'This is the effect of our good feeding, and gentlemen, lest when I am gone, you may be at a loss for an epitaph for me, let me give you one in three words: "He fed fevers."' Graves had made the logical observation that a healthy man starved for weeks became weakened, but that oddly the medical profession expected a man ill with fever to improve when denied food and continuously bled. He attributed many fatalities to this form of therapy and advocated frequent meals of steak, mutton or fowl, washed down with wine and porter.

Corrigan was preaching a similar philosophy on the north side of the city. He disapproved strongly of treatment that weakened and depleted the patient. Discussing a child suffering from episodes of palpitation he commented:

> In some of those cases there is a disposition to bleed from the nose, and the haemorrhage is occasionally very profuse, and this, coupled with pain of the side, which is occasionally present, leads to treatment not calculated to amend the symptoms. The boy is denied animal food. He is sent to the infirmary of the school, and given tartar emetic and bled, or lowered in other ways by purgative or nauseating medicine.

Corrigan's alternative was sea air, sea-bathing, a full diet, wine and iron. He advocated opiates in generous dosage together with local measures to relieve the pain and swelling of the inflamed joints. Whether or not this resulted in much opium addiction is debatable, but at least 'the patient cured by opium has neither bleeding, blistering, nor mercury, to recover from in his convalescence'.

Corrigan's fever reports are characteristic of his style; he holds his readers attention by referring now to one case, then to another:

> You remember the case of Toner. He was admitted on 25th February, on the eighth day of maculated fever, with suffused eyes and dark maculae, his pulse 108, very weak. He was put on wine. Now what was the result? That under the administration of wine, in very large quantities, on the thirteenth day the suffusion of the eyes began to disappear, and, on the sixteenth day, he was convalescent ... But in the case of Matthews in whom the maculae were very dark in colour, and his eyes, too, were congested, sixteen ounces of wine was without effect and blistering had to be resorted to.

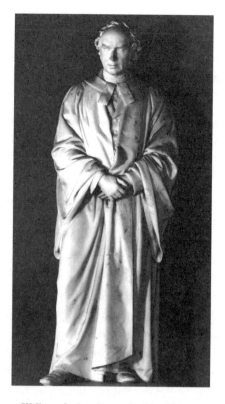

*William Stokes. Statue by John Foley in
the Royal College of Physicians of Ireland (D. Davison).*

William Stokes (1804–1878) differed from other members of the school, in being not only an astute and successful clinician, but also a man of learning with a deep appreciation for the arts. When he returned from Edinburgh to join Graves at the Meath Hospital he brought with him the stethoscope, which caused quite a stir:

> There was much surprise and no little incredulity, with a shade of opposition, shown by sneering, or as we say now, 'chaffing' in its first introduction. The juniors looked at it with amazement, as a thing to gain information by – it so put them in mind of the pop-gun of their school-boy days; the seniors with incredulity … the first instrument of the kind I saw was a piece of timber (elm, I think) three inches in diameter from twelve to fourteen inches long, having a hole drilled through it from top to bottom, no ear-piece, and no attempt at ornamentation. It was amusing to watch the shakes of the head as this bludgeon was passed from hand to hand among the pupils, and to listen to the comments made by them.

Stokes published two papers that earned him eponymous fame. As we have seen he described a form of breathing often seen in terminal illness, which had been previously described by John Cheyne. Stokes's description of this condition now known as 'Cheyne-Stokes respiration' is word perfect:

> The inspirations become each one less deep than the preceding until they are all but imperceptible, and then the state of apparent apnoea (no breathing) occurs. This is at last broken by the faintest possible inspiration, the next effect is a little stronger, until, so to speak, the paroxysm of breathing is at its height, again to subside by a descending scale.

Few could rival him with the stethoscope, but the wise patient having received his diagnostic deliberations, might do best to decline his advice on treatment. In bronchitic children he advocated that the gums should be 'freely and completely divided to allow the teeth to appear'. He supported the common practice of bleeding in most illnesses, but he found that the application of leeches 'applied to the mucous membrane, as near as possible to the epiglottis' was particularly efficacious: 'The child's breathing becomes easier, the face less swelled, and the skin cooler.' Emetics were also considered advantageous: 'I would advise that the medicine should be so exhibited as to produce free vomiting, at least once every three-quarters of an hour,' but he later modified this form of treatment so that it was possible 'to keep up a state of permanent nausea, without vomiting'.

As William Stokes had rescued from obscurity the work of John Cheyne, so too was he to do for his colleague Robert Adams (1796–1875), another member of the Dublin School. In 1846 Stokes published a paper describing how a slow heart could interfere with consciousness, and he drew attention to an earlier paper by Adams in which he had suggested that 'apoplexy must be considered less a disease in itself than symptomatic of one, the organic seat of which was in the heart'. The disease is today known as 'Stokes-Adams' disease' and the loss of consciousness resulting from the slow heart as 'Stokes-Adams attacks'. Apart from these two famous papers, Stokes published many clinical works, among which were two important books – one on disease of the chest, and another on the heart.

In medical education Stokes was ahead of his time:

> The chief, the long-existing, and I grieve to say it, the still prominent evils among us are the neglect of general education, the confounding of instruction with education, and the giving of greater importance to the special training than to the general culture of the student ... Let us emancipate the student, and give him time and opportunity for the cultivation of his mind, so that in his pupillage he shall not be a puppet in the hands of others, but rather a self-relying and reflecting being.

He would be saddened by medical training today, and in particular he would deplore the neglect of the humanities, and the suppression of cultural development with the emergence of the narrow-minded super-specialist: 'Do not be misled by the opinion that a university education will do nothing more than give you a certain proficiency in classical literature, in the study of logics and ethics, or in mathematical or physical science. If it does these things for you, you will be great gainers, for there is no one branch of professional life in which these studies will not prove the most signal help to you.'

The Dublin School's greatest achievement in medical education was the introduction of bedside teaching in the instruction of doctors. Graves and Stokes inculcated this method to generations of their own students and to many from Europe and America while Dominic Corrigan did likewise with no less enthusiasm in the wards of the Hardwicke Hospital. In one of his lectures Corrigan said:

> Let me earnestly impress upon you the absolute necessity of accustoming yourselves to the practical investigation and note-taking of cases ... Is not one glance worth pages of description? Numerous associations fix in your mind, and for ever, the appearance and symptoms of a living case of disease which you have examined, and on which you brought your senses of sight, touch, and hearing, to bear ...

To emphasize this he was fond of quoting the famous French teacher Bichat to his sometimes none-too-eager students: 'You ask me how I have learnt so much. It is because I have read so little. Books are but copies – why have recourse to copies when the originals are before me? My books are the living and the dead: I study these.'

His advice to students on the art of observation in clinical medicine cannot be improved, and though he was speaking of fever of a type not often seen today, his words capture, as few have ever done, the art of clinical observation:

> Let me suppose you now at the bedside of a fever case; stand there quietly, don't disturb the patient, don't at once proceed to examine pulse, or chest, or abdomen, or to put questions. If you do, you may be greatly deceived, for under a sharp or abrupt question a patient may suddenly rouse himself in reply, answer your questions collectedly, and yet die within three hours. Look at your patient as he lies when you enter the ward or sick room; his very posture speaks a language understood by the experienced eye. It is not unusual for the anxious and young resident to draw the earliest attention of the physician in his morning round to some patient who had appeared to him to be in a most dangerous state all night, and for the physician to take a single glance at the patient, and say in reply, 'Never mind him, he is all right; come to the

next case, it is a bad one.' What is the difference between the two? Merely that of posture.

The first patient, or apparently very bad case, had gone through the agitation of crisis during the night, but at morning visit was asleep, lying three-quarters on his side or half on his face, in the posture instinctively chosen to relieve the diaphragm from abdominal pressure, and with muscular strength enough to retain that posture; while beside him lies the serious case, the man who gave no disturbance during the night, who did not complain, but lies on his back without the preservative instinct and without the strength to change it, and with the abdominal viscera like a nightmare on the diaphragm.

Corrigan realized from his own student days that it was possible to study and learn the theory of medicine from textbooks and lectures. He knew that an intelligent student could pass his final examinations without being skilled in clinical technique, without in effect having examined many patients. At this time the final examination comprised an oral exam and usually a written paper. Corrigan saw the deficiency in this assessment of competence. In 1840 he announced a new form of examination for the students of the Richmond:

> We trust to no verbal examination; but for the last four months of the session, commencing at any time after the first of January, we shall, without any previous notice, select cases as we shall deem proper for our purpose on admission into hospital, and require the candidates for our prizes to take those cases, writing down the symptoms, diagnosis, prognosis, and principle treatment, giving each candidate from a quarter to half an hour for his examination of the case; requiring his notes, however, to be written on the spot.

Later even this competitive clinical examination was not in itself enough to satisfy the Richmond teachers as to the quality of their trainees, and Corrigan instigated a term of apprenticeship during which the student would be permitted the opportunity of showing his worth, while at the same time his teachers could assess his development as a doctor. These Victorian teachers were more than a century ahead of their time in advocating continuous assessment rather than examination alone in evaluating medical students.

Corrigan had tasted the elation of success, the satisfaction of achievement; he was also only too well aware of the depression and lassitude of spirit that may come after the routine of years of caring for the ill, and he saw the medical student as having an important role in preventing this all-too-frequent development:

> The physician or surgeon who has under his charge the poor in an hospital, may tire or grow cold in the exercise of his duty, and active diligence in the care of the sick, might, after a time, unconsciously degenerate into the mere

listless routine of going the round of the wards: but surrounded by intelligent pupils his attention to the sick, and his treatment the subject of observation; his opinions and the grounds of his opinions closely scrutinised, his skill tested by the measure of his success on curable cases, by the examination of the dead in incurable affection, the physician or surgeon can never flag in the discharge of his duty; his pride is kept awake, his character is at stake, and the result is, constantly increasing knowledge to himself, the undeviating exercise of humanity and skill towards the poor, and the benefit to society of the diffusion of professional information.

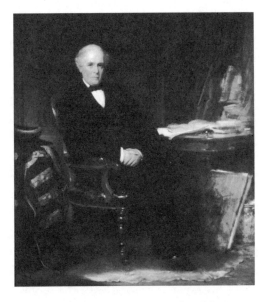

Dominic Corrigan. Statue by John Foley in
the Royal College of Physicians of Ireland (D. Davison).

To many it may come as a surprise to find William Wilde included as a member of the Dublin School. But then, unfortunately, this great Victorian is often remembered only as the father of Oscar, or he is ridiculed and lampooned for his eccentricities and illicit amours. Too often it is forgotten that he was an innovative doctor, an accomplished archaeologist and author of some very fine books on Ireland. Moreover, he and his wife Speranza were Victorian Dublin's most colourful couple. However, let us first put his medical achievements into perspective. None is better qualified to do so than his biographer, the late T.G. Wilson, an ear, nose and throat surgeon, who ranked Wilde as 'one of the two greatest English-speaking aurists of his time', the other referred to being Toynbee. He considered Wilde to be 'almost as brilliant an oculist as he was an aurist'.

William Wilde, the youngest of five children, was born in 1815 in the village of Kilkevin, County Roscommon. His father was a doctor and the son decided to follow in his footsteps. In 1832 'a dark ferrety looking young man below the average size, with retreating chin and a bright roving eye, boarded the coach for Dublin'. He was apprenticed to Abraham Colles and spent four years at Dr Steevens' Hospital, and then went to the Rotunda. After his final exam he collapsed, and Dr Graves was sent for. The astute physician prescribed a glass of strong ale to be taken every hour, and the following morning the dying student was much revived and Graves found him sleeping comfortably. Collapse after finals, particularly in the somewhat Rabelaisian ambiance of the Rotunda Hospital, might be attributable to many causes but Wilson was of the opinion that Wilde had contracted typhus fever. Whatever the cause, he recovered and received his Letters Testimonial from the Royal College of Surgeons in the year of Victoria's accession to the throne, and in the same year we find him the father of his first illegitimate child. The mother was reputedly a Dublin beauty with the unlikely name of Miss Crummles. Sir Henry Marsh and Robert Graves decided that the young surgeon had best leave Dublin for a time, whether for health or social reasons is not clear, and on 24 September 1837 William Wilde sailed down the Solent on the ship *Crusader*, in his charge a patient with consumption on his way to the Holy Land.

During his travels, he developed a keen interest in archaeology, and after witnessing the devastating effects of the eye disease trachoma, so common in Egypt, he decided to specialize in ophthalmology. He published an interesting and successful book of his experiences, and with the profits was able to spend some time on the Continent. In London he was introduced to society by Sir James Clark and Maria Edgeworth. The latter needs no introduction, but Clark is worthy of further mention. 'Poor Clark' as Queen Victoria was later to call him had an unfortunate career. He misdiagnosed pregnancy in Lady Flora Hastings, one of the Queen's maids of honour, when in fact the poor lady was virginal and unfortunately suffering from a malignant abdominal tumour, which later proved fatal. This was a considerable setback to a promising career, but he was retained as the royal physician. When he failed to diagnose typhoid fever as the cause of the Prince Consort's fatal illness, one would have thought his career was at an end. However, Victoria had a deep affection for her physician, and believed that he was more a victim of misfortune than actual incompetence. Whatever his professional shortcomings, he must be judged kindly and with some admiration for the compassion and kindness he showed to the young poet Keats during his last days in Rome.

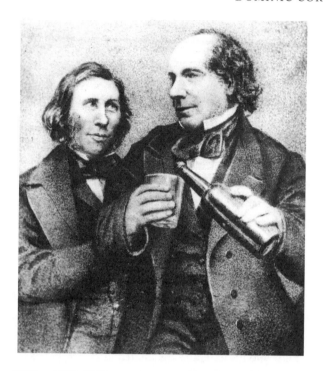

William Wilde (left) *and William Stokes sharing a bottle of beer.*

Here Clark found pleasant apartments for the dying poet and cared for him without expecting or receiving reward. When we remember that there were few at that time who recognized the genius of Keats, least of all the reviewers of the day, we must respect Clark's assessment: 'After all, his expenses will be simple, and he is too noble an animal to be allowed to sink without some sacrifice being made to save him. I wish I were rich enough, his living here should cost him nothing ... I fear there is something operating on his mind ... I feel very much interested in him.' Indeed, there was much troubling the young poet; his mental anguish was if anything greater than his physical suffering – his unfulfilled poetical ambitions and his love for Fanny Brawne.

In the 1840s a young lady, Jane Francesca Elgee, was writing spirited, many would say seditious, prose and poetry for *The Nation*: 'You have never felt the pride, the dignity, the majesty of independence. You could never lift up your head to heaven and glory in the name of Irishmen, for all Europe read the brand of "slavery" upon your brow.' Wilde was fascinated by all this, and in 1851 they were married; a year later William Charles Kinsbury Wills Wilde was born and in 1854 Oscar Fingal O'Flahertie Wills Wilde was introduced to the world.

Wilde, like so many of his contemporaries, was a prodigious worker. Apart from his practice and the running of his hospital, he was editor of the *Dublin Journal of Medicine and Chemical Science*. In 1841 he was appointed assistant census commissioner, a post that involved a vast amount of work, which was rewarded with a knighthood in 1864 when he was aged forty-nine.

In middle life Wilde devoted immense energy to cataloguing the Irish antiquities – a prodigious task, which he performed single-handed, and for which the Royal Academy elected him vice-president and presented to him its highest award, the Cunningham gold medal. He also devoted much time to medical biography and he wrote the fascinating book *The Closing Years of Dean Swift's Life*.

An unfortunate incident was to blight Wilde's career. Sometime in 1854 William Stokes referred Miss Mary Josephine Travers to Wilde with an ear complaint. This twenty-nine year old woman was not beautiful but was of ample proportions, and Wilde found her attractive. We do not know how intimate the relationship became, and can only assume that being a hot-blooded fellow Wilde's intentions, whatever his actions, might not have been altogether platonic. After some years the relationship ended in acrimony. She began a campaign of harassment to both Wilde and his wife, and she invited libel action. The bait was eventually taken and the case became a Victorian scandal of sumptuous proportions. In essence the case was not so much one of libel against Lady Wilde, but rather a trial of Sir William for rape. A thrilled public heard with delight declarations such as, 'I will only say that she went in a maid but out a maid she never departed.'

In the end Lady Wilde was found guilty of libel and fined a farthing, but the costs were substantial. Wilde's career was damaged irreparably and he was a broken man. He retired to his country retreat, Moytura House at Cong in Connemara, where he produced his best-known book – *Lough Corrib*. Three years after the trial the Wildes lost their beloved daughter Isola, and four years later Wilde's two illegitimate daughters died tragically in a fire, an event that affected him greatly. Any happiness in life was now derived from archaeology, and watching the progress of Oscar and Willy through school and university. Sir William died on 19 April 1876 after a long illness. Of his last days we have Oscar's account, which is really a poignant tribute to his mother:

> Before my father died in 1876, he lay ill in bed for many days. And every morning a woman dressed in black and closely veiled used to come to our house in Merrion Square, and unhindered by my mother, or anyone else used to walk straight up stairs to Sir William's bedroom and sit down at the head of his bed and to sit there all day, without ever speaking a word or once raising her veil. She took no notice of anybody in the room; and nobody paid any

attention to her. Not one woman in a thousand would have tolerated her presence, but my mother allowed it because she knew that my father loved the woman and felt that it must be a joy and comfort to have her there by his dying bed. And I am sure that she did right not to grudge that last happiness to a man who was about to die, and I am sure that my father understood her indifference, understood that it was not because she did not love him that she permitted her rival's presence, but because she loved him very much, and died with his heart full of gratitude and affection for her.

The life of the Dublin School of medicine was brief, but its light had burned so brightly that it reached across the world. Corrigan was not unaware of the rise of the School: 'The Irish school of medicine and surgery is, if I am not mistaken, exerting a silent but deeply spreading influence upon society, an influence which is beneficial, and which will I hope be lasting.' He was proud especially of its international influence:

> Until lately this country may be said to have been unknown, or known only to be misrepresented. Latterly foreigners from all parts of Europe of high mental acquirements have visited us, and their numbers each year are increasing; … and if the beacon of knowledge is once more to burn as pre-eminently brightly in my native country, as tradition says it once did, the honour of re-lighting will assuredly belong to my own profession.

The Dublin School began somewhere around 1830 and lasted scarcely fifty years. Its success was dependent foremost on the extraordinary energies and talents of its main progenitors, Graves, Stokes and Corrigan. Others of ability were to follow but they failed to sustain the spirit of the School. We may well wonder why so vibrant a movement was permitted to decay. The conditions in which subsequent generations practised were not substantially different to those of the mid-nineteenth century; there were the same hospitals, with the addition of some new ones; there were more doctors and nursing improved greatly; a limited amount of money for research became available whereas there had been no provision for research funding in Victorian Ireland; the government participated in health care not always acting in the best interests of the sick, but nonetheless, augmenting greatly the voluntary support on which mid-nineteenth-century medicine depended.

And yet the School disappeared. Its *raison d'être* was its iconoclasm, which was fuelled from without rather than within Ireland. The members of the School competed with and enjoyed the company of the European leaders of medicine; their ideals and their standards were pitched well above the mediocrity to which Ireland, through complacency and an insular philosophy, is prepared often from unawareness of anything better, to tolerate. Had later generations been prepared to seek and absorb the influence of European and American medicine, the School might have survived, and Irish medicine might have been saved from a period of stagnation and apathy from which it only now shows some feeble signs of emerging. If today's medical profession is to be enriched from a study of the rise and rapid decline of the Dublin School, it will be by the realization that its future lies not within the narrow confines of the island that is Ireland, but beyond in the broader intellectualism of international science.

Irish Doctors and Literature

THOUGH I SPENT most of my life as a consultant cardiologist in The Charitable Infirmary (and latterly in Beaumont Hospital, which comprises The Charitable Infirmary and the Richmond Hospitals), it is fair to say that my most enduring memories and affection are anchored in the Richmond Hospital. I had, after all, spent much of my childhood there accompanying my father to the hospital as he went on his Sunday rounds. Then it was my teaching hospital, where I spent my student residency days and later worked as a junior doctor, then on my return to Ireland from training in England as a locum physician. The essay, based on a chapter entitled 'Let Verse and Humour be Our Music'[22] attempts to capture the 'character' of the Richmond Hospital. The ethos of the hospital emanated, I think, from a collective sense of impotence in the face of suffering, and an appreciation of the excessive expectation of society on the 'doctor' to be able to alleviate that suffering. The inability of the medical profession to match the demands of the public in its charge could be faced by despondency or by a realism tempered with humour and art.

This, I believe, was what the Richmond offered to me as student and later as a doctor. I could and must recount sometime the legacy of fond memories these men bequeathed to me. I knew many of the doctors with literary interests in this essay; one in particular springs to mind. I persuaded Daragh Smith to give a talk about his student days some forty years on and I recall just one gem from his lively discourse. Daragh, wishing to convey to his listeners the power of a local parish curate about to address his parish on the controversial issue of donations to the Church during the depression of the 1950s, described how the curate, on entering the sunlit church, immediately established his God-given authority by 'hanging his cloak on a sunbeam' before ascending to the pulpit.

Let Verse and Humour Be Our Music, 1988

ST LAURENCE'S HOSPITAL, more often known as the Richmond Hospital, where I walked the wards as a student and later as a member of the staff, has a literary legacy that is often overlooked.

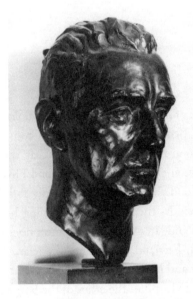

*Oliver St John Gogarty. Bronze bust
by Fife Waters (courtesy Meath Hospital).*

When Oliver St John Gogarty died in New York in 1957, Dublin medicine lost one of its most colourful and talented personalities. Though Gogarty was not always popular among his colleagues, none could deny the scope of his talent and the influence he exerted on Irish life and politics. Ulick O'Connor, in his masterful biography of Gogarty, puts his diverse achievements thus:

> W.B. Yeats in his preface to the *Oxford Book of Modern Verse*, refers to Oliver
> St. John Gogarty as 'one of the great lyric poets of the age'. Asquith called

Gogarty the wittiest man in London. Edward Shanks thought his conversation had the flavour of Wilde's. Gogarty was also a skilful surgeon, an aviator, a senator, a playwright, a champion athlete and swimmer. When Professor Mario Rossi, an Italian authority on Swift and Berkeley, met Gogarty in the thirties he felt he was in the presence of a figure out of the Renaissance, *l'uomo universale*, the 'all-sided man'.

One may quibble perhaps about Gogarty's skill as a surgeon, but when he is judged in the context of his time he is seen as a competent, if not brilliant, ENT surgeon with innovative flair, who introduced Bruning's bronchoscope to Dublin from Vienna. His literary achievements, obviously more substantial than his medical ones, are not so easily assessed. Gogarty once wrote of Browning, 'He does not write poetry, but his prose pulsates.' One might state exactly the opposite for Gogarty; he wrote some perfect poetry but his prose, of which there is much, was often turgid, clumsy and lacking the form that would have benefitted from the discipline he applied so successfully to his poetry. This said, his autobiographical prose works do give an interesting insight into his life as a leading member of the medical profession and the literati of Dublin in the early twentieth century.

Gogarty did medicine, like so many before and after him, simply because there was 'doctoring' in the family. His grandfather and father had both been doctors. His mother wished to have him registered in the Catholic Medical School in Cecilia Street, but a lack of gentlemanly courtesy by the registrar Ambrose Birmingham made her take her young charge across the river to Trinity College, where the Provost, Dr Anthony Traill, made a much more favourable impression. She admonished her son after this experience: 'Now that you are entered among gentlemen I hope you never forget to behave like one.'

Though Gogarty may never have let his mother down by being ungentlemanly, he did throw himself into student life with an ardour of which mamma could hardly have approved. Poetry and literature vied with medicine for his intellectual attention, with women, cycling and the congenial ambience of literary Dublin being distractions that he found difficult to resist. His medical apprenticeship occupied ten leisurely years during which time he became renowned, not only in Dublin but also in Oxford, for his wit and genial company. Picture George Moore and W.B. Yeats after dinner one evening discussing animatedly the composition of the last line of Gogarty's latest limerick:

> There was a young man from St Johns
> Who wanted to roger the swans.
> 'On no!' said the porter,

'Oblige with my daughter,
For the birds are reserved for the dons.'

Gogarty's student attachment was to the Richmond Hospital. From his comments on Dublin hospitals we can take it that he would have mixed feelings on the
recent closure of so many of these institutions:

There are nineteen hospitals in Dublin, and all of them are unmergeable into
one …There is a greater vested interest in disease than in Guinness's Brewery.
This explains why it would give rise to far more trouble than it is worth to
run the nineteen into one. Besides the unemployment it would create and the
disease it would end! Disease is not always a heart-breaking and melancholy
affair, as might be supposed. Where there are so many hospitals for so small
a city; diseases thin out as it were in proportion to their deadliness; they tend
to become chronic and tolerable.

Gogarty also turned his wit on the religious intolerance that once so dominated our hospitals, and the influence of which is clearly palpable to this day:

Disease in Dublin is a *modus vivendi* and it therefore assumes a religious
aspect. There are Protestant, Catholic and Presbyterian diseases in Dublin.
The Adelaide; Sir Patrick Dun's; the City of Dublin, commonly called Baggot
Street Hospital; the Meath; and Stevens (sic); these are all Protestant hospitals. Stevens (sic) deals largely with police 'who also serve' but are liable to
contract venereal disease while standing and waiting – on point duty! In the
Adelaide only respectable diseases are treated.

The Richmond in Gogarty's student days seemed to achieve something ap-
proaching a religious balance: 'The Richmond has more knights and Presbyte-
rians than all the other hospitals in the town. There were Sir Thornley Stoker, his
brother-in-law Sir William Thomson, and Sir Thomas Myles: Protestants all. The
Catholic balance consisted of Dr Coleman and Dr O'Carroll; Sir Conway Dwyer
was afterwards introduced.'

Gogarty's life as a student was full and enjoyable. Though not successful in
passing his medical exams, he was developing his intellect in other ways, not least
in poetry – at Oxford he came second to his friend George Bell in the Newdigate
Prize. Back in Dublin however, the exams were causing problems and even the
muse failed to provide the inspiration needed to compensate for a memory scarce
in medical knowledge:

'I'm going to swerve,'
Said the lingual nerve.
'Well be sure you avoid,'

Said the pterygoid,
'Myself and the ramus
When passing between us.'
'Oh you'll be bucked,'
Said Wharton's duct,
'When you land in the kip
At the tongue's top tip.'

Drinking in these past days was not always confined to Dublin's pubs, more frequent by far than the lazar houses, which Gogarty found so excessive. The medical student's preference was often for the cosier atmosphere of the kips of Nightown, situated in the vicinity of Railway Street and Tyrone Street. Here, as O'Connor explains with what may be a naivety born out of respect for his subject, a tired student could drink all night without having to absent himself on the felicity upstairs. 'This was one of the advantages of the place for medical students whose duties involved their being abroad at hours when it was difficult to obtain refreshment elsewhere.' Gogarty has recorded the activities of the Kips, the only licensed brothel area in the then United Kingdom, in the poem 'The Hay Hotel':

There is a window stuffed with hay
Like Herbage in an oven cast;
And there we came at break of day
To soothe ourselves with light repast:
And men who worked before the mast
And drunken girls delectable;
A future symbol of our past
You'll maybe, find the Hay Hotel.

Where is Piano Mary say,
Who dwelt where Hell's Gates leave the street,
And all the tunes she used to play
Along your spine beneath the sheet?
She was a morsel passing sweet
And warmer than the gates of hell
Who tunes her now between the feet
Go ask them at the Hay Hotel.
    L'ENVOI
Nay; never ask this week, fair Lord.
If, where they are now, all goes well,
So much depends on bed and board
They give them in the Hay Hotel.

Gogarty's teachers at the Richmond were Sir Thomas Myles, Sir Robert Woods, Sir William Thomson, Sir Thornley Stoker, surgeons all, and Dr 'Jock' O'Carroll, a physician much beloved by students and patients. Little is remembered today of these personalities.

Of William Thomson, Gogarty had this to say: 'He was one of those whose grandeur depends on silence. If a grand manner could cure disease, Sir William would be the world's benefactor.'

Thomas Myles, a handsome man who indulged in boxing, yachting and reading Shakespeare, appealed greatly to young Gogarty. He once paused before performing 'a certain operation performed exclusively on males' to remark, 'There is a divinity that shapes our ends.' Sir Thomas enlivened clinical teaching with frequent references to Shakespeare; a syphilitic sailor presented him with a magnificent opportunity:

> He has braved the arctic night and he has heard the thunder of the breaking ice. He has seen the great whale shouldering off the seas as he comes to the surface. Ah, but gentlemen, the shore has its dangers as great, if not greater, than the deep and the ways of women can be deadlier than the sea; some dalliance, some little sport with Amaryllis in the shade, some entanglement with Neaera's hair, and the lurking principle entered in then that appears on the surface twenty years later.

Sir Robert Woods, ear, nose and throat surgeon, was to influence Gogarty to follow in his footsteps. Indeed when Gogarty later returned from Vienna after training under Chiari and Hajek, Woods assured his future prospects with the remark: 'There will be enough in my back-wash, Gogarty, to keep you going for the rest of your life.'

William Thornley Stoker, brother of Bram, the author of *Dracula*, was a well-known surgeon whose interest outside medicine was collecting antiques. Gogarty, who later became his close friend, attributed Stoker's collection to the maladies he treated: 'The Aubusson carpet in the drawing-room represents a hernia, the Ming Cloisonne a floating kidney, the Buhl cabinet his opinion of an enlarged liver, the Renaissance bronze on the landing, a set of gall-stones.'

O'Connor makes what is probably a valid statement in his biography of Gogarty: 'The spectacle of suffering humanity brought out in him a kindness that those who knew only the forked-tongue Gogarty of the dining table and salon could never have suspected.' In support of this view we may merely note that if Gogarty had not felt the compassion for suffering that is a prerequisite to being a good doctor, he would have failed to record such sentiments, much less write a drama, *Blight*, which opened in the Abbey Theatre in 1917. (This play, described as 'the tragedy of Dublin – the horrible, terrible, creeping crawling spectre that haunts the slumdom of the capital of Ireland', was important not only as a social statement, but as a landmark in dramatic literature that marked the advent of the 'slum play' that was later to be developed by O'Casey.) Gogarty's sense of compassion is further exemplified in his awareness of the suffering to which doctors are continuously exposed and the effects that this may have on a sensitive mind.

The realities of the less attractive side of a medical career are strongly enunciated in Jock O'Carroll's discourse to his students in the Richmond, as penned by Gogarty in *Tumbling in the Hay*:

> Turn back now if you are not prepared and resigned to devote your lives to the contemplation of pain, suffering and squalor. For realize that it is not with athletes that you will be consorting, but with the dying and the diseased. The sunny days will not be yours any longer but days in the crowded dispensaries, the camp of the miner or of the soldier where, unarmed, you must render service in the very foremost positions. It is in the darkened pathological department of some institution that you, some of you, will spend your lives in tireless investigation of that microcosmic world which holds more numerous and more dangerous enemies of man than the deep. Your faces will alter. You will lose your youthful smirks; for, in the end, your ceaseless traffic with suffering will reflect itself in grave lines upon your countenance. Your outlook on life will have none of the deception that is the unconscious support of the layman: to you all life will appear in transit, and you will see with clear and undeceived vision the different stages of its devolution and its indivertible path to the grave. You will see those sightless forces, the pull of gravity, the pull of the grave that never lets up for one moment, draw down the cheeks and the corners of the mouth and bend the back until you behold beauty abashed and life itself caricatured in the spectacle of the living looking down on the sod as if to find a grave.

Gogarty's compassion is also reflected in his poetry. One poem, 'All the Pictures', which may not be perfect in its composition, does convey the sadness doctor experiences in the face of hopelessness, and the admiration inspired by the stoicism of a patient. The poem was written as a tribute to a patient who, hearing the news that there was no hope for him, replied, 'I have seen all the pictures.'

> I told him he would soon be dead.
> 'I have seen all the pictures,' said
> My patient. 'And I do not care.'
> What could a doctor do but stare

In admiration half amused
Because the fearless fellow used
'The pictures' as a metaphor,
And was the first to use it for
Life which he could no longer feel
But only see it as a reel?
Was he not right to be resigned
To the sad wisdom of his mind?
Who wants to live when Life's a sight
Shut from the inner senses quite;
When listless heart and cynic mind
Are closed within a callous rind;
When April with its secret green
Is felt no more but only seen,
And Summer with its dusky meadows
Is no more than a play of shadows;
And Autumn's garish oriflamme
Fades like a flickering skiagram,
And all one's fiends are gone, or seem
Shadows of dream beyond a dream?
And woman's love not any mo,
Oh, surely then 'tis time to go
And join the shades that make the Show!

John Hackett Pollock, born in 1887, was assistant pathologist to the Richmond Hospital, where he is best remembered for his Saturday morning demonstrations on the museum's pathological specimens. A gentle, kindly man, who when aroused could be acerbic in his comments, he was attracted more to literature than to medicine. Pollock published at least nineteen books, many under the pseudonym An Philibín. His writing deserves reappraisal. He wrote poetry and criticism, but his greatest literary contribution was as a novelist. Though he showed, in his criticism of Yeats, astute appreciation of the poetic method, his own verse tends to lack the 'spare severity and approach to that stern colour, delicate line and secret discipline', he so much admired in Yeats to whom he paid 'the supreme compliment of finding no comparison with any other English poet possible'. In Pollock's poem 'Dublin', the social conscience of the doctor, as in Gogarty's 'Blight', is again evident.

Pollock's novel, *Peter and Paul* (1933), almost perfect in its construction and only failing in the excesses of the prologue to its tragic conclusion, is as fine a depiction of the conflicting religious and social influences in Dublin in the first twenty years of the last century as has been written. The drama of the tragedy that is *Peter and Paul* might have had greater impact on the stage but Pollock, who was not greatly taken by Yeats's efforts on behalf of national drama, decided no doubt to leave the theatre aside.

In *Peter and Paul* there is, as inevitably there must be in any Irish drama, a gentle thread of wry humour. In one scene the unambitious gauche dispensary doctor from Durrow, Dr Nicholas Kilfeather, visits his one-time rival for honours at medical school, who is now flourishing in wealthy ostentation as a consultant on Fitzwilliam Square.

Pollock had an eye for the beauty around him and the pastoral tranquillity of the Dublin suburbs is captured more than once in *Peter and Paul*:

He travelled by train to Sutton, where he boarded the Summit tram, absorbing the beauty of the locality, visited for the first time. To the north stretched the silver curves of Portmarnock, Malahide and Donabate, washed by a sea of indigo; before him rose Shiel Martin and Ben Edar, whence came the warm almondy smell of blossoming whin; while southward lay the Dublin Bay, the entire indented coastline from Wicklow Head to the city topped by the upcast peaks and spurs of violet hill. He descended from the tram at the little thatched cottage entitled 'Baily Post Office', rather at a loss, half expecting to be met by someone of his acquaintance.

Though the physician in Pollock rarely intrudes in his writing, there are those occasions when the novelist in him draws, as all novelists do, on life's own store of experience. The physician in so doing is particularly advantaged in this regard in portraying disease. In *Peter and Paul*, Pollock paints a masterly picture of middle-aged depression:

'It's difficult to translate intimate personal feelings and nuances into words,' began Dardis slowly, 'and any terms I may use are merely verbal approxima-tions to the actual condition. This state of mind has been developing slowly for some time past, and lately appears to be heading for some kind of crisis … it commenced with a profound sense of futility in every feature of my work, which subsequently extended to the simplest necessary details of every-day life … it has now become so fixed that I frequently ask myself is there any real, fundamental necessity, for getting up say, in the morning, or sitting down to dinner … I am oppressed also by a profound conviction of my own superfluity in the scheme of things; and this symptom has more than once threatened to develop into the more positive idea that I am not merely unnecessary, but possibly an actual impediment to others more competent for life than myself … Lately what is most distressing is a ghastly sensation of inhabiting a world peopled by masked automations ... horrible robots who have no more qualification for natural wholesome existence than I possess ... There isn't anything else to tell you,' he concluded, 'except that I'm not sleeping properly for a considerable time past.'

Pollock, the pathologist, has left little other than some pleasant anecdotal memories; Pollock, the writer, has bequeathed a rich legacy worthy of reappraisal. He died in December 1964.

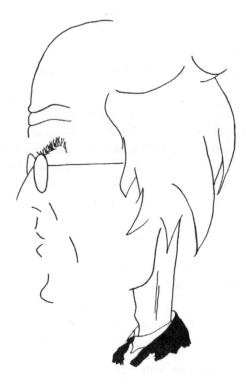

John Pollock.

Jack Widdess, physician, historian, man of letters, bibliophile and kindly mentor to aspiring historians, wrote the histories of four medical institutions – *The Royal College of Surgeons in Ireland and its Medical School* was first published in 1949 (a revised edition was published in 1967), and a *History of the Royal College of Physicians of Ireland* appeared in 1963; for the two hundred and fiftieth anniversary of The Charitable Infirmary in 1968, he edited *The Charitable Infirmary, Jervis Street, 1718–1968*, and in 1972 wrote *The Richmond, Whitworth and Hardwicke Hospitals: St Laurence's, Dublin 1772–1972*, to commemorate that institution's bicentenary.

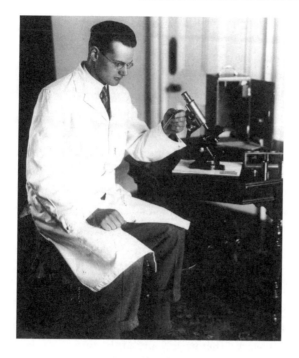

J.D.H. Widdess.

Jack Widdess was obsessional, sometimes to the point of annoyance, and yet it was this obdurate attention to detail that makes his historical legacy so valuable. He was not, however, suited to the discipline of verbal communication, which is not to say that he could resist the opportunity to expound on his favourite topic. The time constraints of mere fractions of hours were nothing to him when dealing with centuries of fact, and yet he was able to distil his researches and avoid any tediousness in his writing. His style was lively and entertaining and, without compromising historical accuracy, he was able to blend the humour and sadness of history with a subtlety that was most attractive. He was not a stimulating lecturer in biology, and one suspects that he did not believe in didactic lectures, whereas his demonstrations on the subjects were interesting and memorable.

In the seventies Jack was one of a group whose lunchtime conversation in the dining-room of the 'Convent' in the Richmond was usually interesting and sometimes memorable. Here the rhythm 'The Sea Baboon' was discussed with the same intensity as the latest production of *The Valkyrie* at Bayreuth, and, while one group expounded on fly-fishing in the west of Ireland, another might be heard analysing the semantic ingeniousness of a senior Garda's pronouncement that the city was being overrun, not so much by prostitutes, but by 'little whoreens'. It was in this ambiance that Jack could give rein to a capricious and, at times, mischievous humour, often the more remarkable for a bawdiness that emanated from a deceptively saturnine countenance.

Daragh Smith, who once graced the student quarters of the Richmond in the thirties, has left in the verse of his *Dissecting Room Ballads* an irreverent glimpse of an irreverent age. These *Ballads* capture in a unique way a period of Dublin medical life that has passed into the mists of time. For all their licentiousness, these verses from the dead-room express an innocence that cannot be submerged in their content. Medical students throughout time have professed more than an academic interest in matters carnal. A libidinous zest for life, whether due to close companionship with death, a premature awareness of the frailty of human existence, or merely a consequence of a prolonged, if not absolute celibacy (a state breached only by a stroke of rare fortune in Dublin of the thirties), is a characteristic of the Aesculapian disciple.

The *Ballads* mark a transitional phase in the mores of the Dublin medical student. Gone are the kips of Annie Mack and May Oblong in Monto with their 'drunken girls delectable' so celebrated in prose by Joyce, and lamented in their passing by Gogarty. The promiscuity of the twenties was being replaced by the inhibitive chastity that was to characterize the forties and fifties. The *Ballads* emanate something of the extremes of both eras. So we find irreverence going hand-in-hand with innocence, as is the case so often with life. And perhaps that is how we should take the *Ballads*, as a hedonistic youthful expression of existence that takes the present for what it is and cares not a damn for an uncertain future.

The *Ballads* were known verbatim by all students of the Richmond (and many more besides) during the middle decades of the century and senior members of staff have been known to discuss at great length the correct rendering of 'Brian Boru's French Letter' or the syntax of 'The Sea Baboon'.

BRIAN BORU'S FRENCH LETTER

I was up to my oxters in turf mould
At my turf contract down in the bog
When my slane chanced to strike against something
Like a stone, or a lump of a log.

'Twas a box of the finest bogoak, Sir,
And I wondered just what it might hide
So I muttered 'Well – bugger the fairies!'
And I took a wee look, Sir, inside.

I suppose now, you'll scarcely believe me
It's almost too good to be true
'Twas an *Ancient Irish French Letter*
A relic of Brian Boru!

'Twas an ancient Irish French letter
Made of elk skin, and just a foot tall.
And a little gold tag at the bottom
Gave his name, and his stud fee, and all.

And my mind flittered back through the ages
To the time of that sturdy old Celt.
There was Granuaile up on the bedstead
And Brian Boru in his pelt.

And I heard him remark rather firmly
'Listen here now, we must get this right,
Though you did have your own way last night Dear
It's the hairy side outwards tonight.'

THE SEA BABOON

Oh why are the wild waves fleckt wi' blood
And the sea shore stained with red?
Oh hark The Tale of the Sea Baboon –
The tale of a race now dead!

The last of his race was the Sea Baboon,
Huge, and black with an oily skin,
And his penis pink and his foreskin too
Had an undulant dorsal fin.

Of a sudden a thought struck the Sea Baboon
And he closed his jaws with a snap!
And he looked at his balls – his hairy balls
Like a bear curled up in his lap.

And then into the sea dashed the Sea Baboon,
Lust, passion had entered his soul
For the spring had come to that solitary beast
And he longed, yes he longed – for his Hole!

A female shark came swimming along
A quiet elderly dame
And he ambled up and accosted her
With never a thought of shame!

And he caught her tail as she whisked away
(Oh vile, unnatural crime!)
She yielded, and there on the ocean bed
They worked away for a while.

This served to whet his appetite –
He next had a slim young whale;
Then a couple more sharks and as yet no sign
Of his prowess beginning to fail.

Look! What is that swift and graceful form?
That alluring shade of grey!
'We'll have one more' says the Sea Baboon
'Then we'll chuck it and call it a day.'

But alas, the Submarine, U.6.3.
Its propeller whirrs apace!
And it cut off the balls of the Sea Baboon
The last pair of BALLS in the RACE.

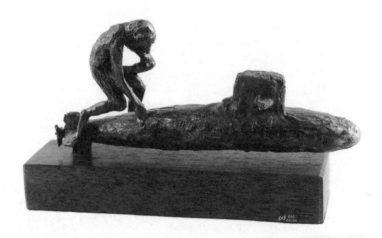

*The Sea Baboon. Bronze sculpture by Pat Dolan, presented
to Daragh Smith in the Park Hotel, Virginia, on 20 September 1985.*

Dom Peter Flood

I FIRST HEARD of the legendary J.C. Flood from my father, and when I joined the staff of The Charitable Infirmary I met some of his contemporaries who were able to tell me more of this enigmatic misogynist and generally much unloved figure. Des Murray, a surgeon, recounted how he learned with delight that Flood, who was a surgeon on the staff of The Charitable Infirmary, announced that he was going to Ealing Abbey to take Holy Orders. He also described his bitter disappointment some months later on entering the hall of the hospital to see the back of a tonsured head that announced Flood's return. However, happily – at least for Murray – this lapse was temporary and the 'call of God' soon reclaimed him permanently for Ealing Abbey.

However, this was not to be Murray's last encounter with Flood. Tony Walsh, another surgeon in the hospital, arranged to be married in Ealing Abbey with Flood as the chief celebrant; as Flood came down the aisle with his troop of concelebrants he passed Murray, who was having some difficulty undoing the bow that graced the wedding ceremony programme, and threw him the aside: 'Having difficulty as always, Murray, with your sutures.' I decided that I had better see for myself on what Flood's notoriety was founded and so I visited him at Ealing Abby in 1976. I wrote the essay 'Lunch at Ealing Abbey' after his death in 1978.[23]

Lunch at Ealing Abbey, 1979

J.C. FLOOD has been, for me, a legend for as far back as I can remember. My father had entertained many a medical student with ribald anecdotes of his caustic wit and, later, Flood's contemporaries were to speak to me with some awe of a man who had more than a little influence on Dublin medicine for many years. Then there were the stories from UCD of the oratorical battles he waged at the L& H in the course of acquiring one of his many degrees at Earlsfort Terrace. When I was appointed to the staff of The Charitable Infirmary, I set off for Ealing Abbey to see if the myth was a reality. As I sat in the parlour awaiting this infamous misogynist, who it was said had declared women to be not only physically inferior but mentally subordinate to the male, I wished that the present I carried for my wife did not have *Just Jane Maternity Boutique* emblazoned across its wrapping. The door burst open and there, in flowing robe, erect, and looking a little like Alastair Sim in an opera cloak, was Dom Peter, who looked me straight in the eye and said:

> And so you're Doctor O'Brien of Dublin – welcome. You are to succeed Tommy Ryan, who I had appointed to Jervis Street, and as yours was a Charter appointment every member of the Board of Governors, myself included, had a vote. But, of course, it is nothing like the old days when there were some 200 governors, all of whom had to be approached personally if one was to succeed, and that meant days loitering around hospital corridors and kicking the sawdust from the portals of many a pub door. And in the end they always did what Reverend Mother said, but you had to do it, nonetheless – very tiresome.

As we made our way towards the refectory for lunch, he apologized for the comforts of carpeting and central heating, lamenting, 'Progress is irresistible, and these young fellows will have their way.' He warned me that conversation was forbidden during lunch, 'a good thing in my opinion as it saves a lot of tiresome chatter, and besides only the Irish and the French are capable of good conversation, and there are no other representatives of either nation here'.

After lunch, he recalled the old days when the likes of Johnny McArdle 'would be brought by special CIE train (complete with nurse), as if a royal personage, to the home of a country dignitary so that the good gentleman might die with the best possible people about him'. One day when conducting his outpatients according to his usual policy – new patients first, then women and children, and finally men – a couple of Jim Larkin's union members demanded immediate attention, warning that if they were not seen Big Jim would hear about it; faced with Flood's refusal to change his policy the pair marched off in the direction of Liberty Hall, but Flood motored to the same establishment ahead of them and, bursting unannounced into Larkin's office, delivered a stern caveat that if Larkin's union ever attempted to dictate to him – Surgeon Flood – trouble of indescribable magnitude would ensue. He compared Larkin in appearance to Paisley, whose unfortunate parish priest Flood had admonished for failing in his duty to see that Paisley's children were reared as Catholics, and not only that, he had advised Cardinal Conway to give Paisley status as 'a religious leader in the North of Ireland, so that two great moderating religious leaders might carry the people over their differences'.

He had been fond of Dublin: 'The Liffeyside houses gave to Dublin its continental atmosphere, and it was a tragic mistake to pull down so many. There is the most beautiful view of the city from one bed in St Patrick's ward, from where at sunset can be seen Christ Church Cathedral throwing its shadow over the old part of Dublin and the Liffey – I always said I would die in that bed'. He chuckled at the thought. 'I moved heaven and earth to get theatres built on the top floor of Jervis Street, but the Governors turned it down because in the event of fire water could not be pumped to that height. I told them to get better pumps, but they did not listen. Of course, the theatres are on the rooftop now.'

Flood feared that standards in medicine were deteriorating:

There is no vocation left in medicine. I insisted on seeing my patients personally on the first post-operative day, even if that was a Sunday, and if I ever went to see a private patient on a Sunday, I would also make a point of seeing my public patients. If you are ever having an operation, never leave it later than Wednesday, otherwise the entire staff will be golfing when your post-operative complications set in. I could forgive one of my staff making a mistake provided I was informed at a stage when corrective action was possible, but I would dismiss without hesitation the doctor who tried to cover up, because then he or she is not acting in the patient's interest.

I was in hospital recently myself having a prostatectomy, and quite enjoyed it. I refused all visitors. Things have not changed much except there are a lot of black people, including one charming black maid of great cultural worth – we talked for hours on China and she from darkest Africa. I did welcome one thing though; on recovering from anaesthesia, the surgeon said – 'All is well, the operation was a success.' Very comforting that; how often we forget to tell the patient the result of the operation, and they are afraid to ask.

Actually my medical career only ended comparatively recently – I was sacked as infirmarian to the Abbey; they said I refused to give them aspirin and paracetamol, which is not quite true, although I would certainly have refused if they had asked. I will not be told by a patient what I should prescribe, and anyway aspirin causes gastric ulceration and paracetamol is broken down to phenacetin causing kidney disease; these drugs should be controlled by prescription.

I asked him if there was truth in the story that after Leonard Abrahamson had presented to the Academy a complicated case of rheumatoid arthritis treated over many years with gold, Flood had asked, 'Can the learned professor tell us if, after the good lady's demise, he managed to recover the gold?' He laughed quite heartily at this, but said he did not think it was true, adding that whoever had concocted it had done a good job. I told him that his was not to be the last laugh, and that to 'the Abe' was attributed the classic mot, 'Flood has more degrees than a thermometer without the same capacity for registering warmth.' He also laughed at this, but not with much enthusiasm, and went on to tell me that he had acquired another degree since then – a doctorate in canon law during his fourteen years as professor of moral theology in Rome; he had found this more difficult than all the others put together, namely, an MB, M.Ch., membership of King's Inns, and a BA in economics and in languages. I asked him why he had acquired so many degrees and he told me that some, such as economics and law, were of necessity as he had 'commercial interests', but there was more to it than that: 'I never talk about anything unless I know my subject extremely well. If I don't know anything about something, I say nothing. Simple, is it not? A pity everybody doesn't follow suit.'

He went on to discuss the art of preaching:

> When I am giving a lecture to seminarians, I tell them of the recently ordained priest giving his first sermon, which he prepares and rehearses with great care and finally delivers with reasonable assurance, if a little hesitantly and shyly, but this is forgiven because everybody knows it is his first sermon; he then puts the text of the sermon in a box, and he does likewise with subsequent sermons, and when, forty years later, he is called upon to preach on the same topic, he roots around in the box, finds the appropriate sermon and delivers it again.

Flood banged his fist on the table in rage declaring, 'I say to them, what that ignorant man has done is to state to his audience that he has leaned nothing in forty years – he has denied them the experience of forty years – isn't that an awful thought? But, of course, these young fellows don't listen to me – they will all do exactly what I tell them not to do.'

We discussed cardiology for a while – a short while.

> Actually, I have very little time for cardiologists, although I do attend one regularly; an extremely nice chap, Dublin of course; perhaps you know him. Got quite a bright wife too, I believe. Yes, he gives me tablets, a new thing

called a-something-blocker. He took me off aldomet, which had suited me quite well for many years without, I might add, lowering my blood pressure one whit, but of course, the Inderal has no effect either. I told Walter, I said to him, there is no point in giving me anything, all will be useless, but he insisted on my taking these, telling me that they were tiny and that I would hardly notice them. I reminded him that I could give him cyanide, which he would hardly notice either, apart from the result, at which stage, of course, his observations would be of little avail. Anyway, I take them for Walter, at least, occasionally when I remember them. Yes, I really have very little time for cardiologists. A friend of mine, a doctor, phoned me one day from the London Clinic to say he was dying and would not last very long and could I come to see him – quickly, as he might not be able to wait.

So, of course, off I went, but was told at the reception desk that he was critically ill and was not being permitted visitors. Ignoring these protestations, I proceeded up the stairs to his room, where another nurse informed me that the presence of a visitor would most surely precipitate the doctor's departure. Sweeping her aside, I entered the room where I found my friend looking remarkably fit, definitely not a dying man, even I could tell that, but he assured me that he was on the way out and that time was short. I discussed some of his many family problems, for which he blamed himself. I then told him to get up, and giving him my hand I helped him from his death-bed, assisted him to dress, and on leaving the room I informed the horror-stricken nurse that the patient was now ready for discharge, and would she be so kind as to inform his consultant cardiologist that his patient was cured.

With a mischievous glance, he forecast my future:

So, you're going to listen to hearts for the rest of your life, tut, tut! I suppose it could be worse. You hear nothing really, nobody at the bedside believes you've heard anything regardless of what you say. They just keep talking while you listen. It's very difficult to be flamboyant with a stethoscope, very difficult to have style, but I suppose you'll get new machinery, something bigger and better than the ECG – play around with it for a while and then discard it. Mind you, it's very difficult to be an eccentric character in medicine nowadays – you are all paid too well, and when you are well paid there is no need to have flair. Of course, the surgeon has a much better chance, a knife is much more theatrical than a stethoscope, and then there's all the dressing up to go with it. I suppose they even wear make-up nowadays.

I ventured that Gogarty had flair, but he found this suggestion as unpleasant as the memory of that contemporary wit:

Perhaps he was good at ENT surgery, but I would not be in a position to judge; he was a complete chancer, a phoney, and a show-off – always a sign of weakness in a man. I suppose his swans have disappeared from the Liffey – ran from his own shadow, heh, heh! Joyce had his measure as Buck Mulligan, but then Joyce had great power of character description before he went mad and wrote that last tome of mumbo-jumbo. Imagine that fellow Gogarty being called in one afternoon to operate on a wealthy private patient who, lying terrified on the table, sees this breathless fool arriving late, declare as he took two pistols from his coat pockets, 'I am a marked man' – really shameless showmanship, tut, tut!

He asked about my family, and on learning that I had one son and one of unknown gender on the way, commented with some feeling:

That's nice, great to watch them growing up. I would like to have had ten boys and ten girls – came from a large family myself – but, of course, having taken orders this wasn't possible. Still, I do have my spiritual children, a number of young seminarians, very devoted, treat me much like a father, same sort of relationship, better in a lot of ways – I can choose them.

I served for fourteen years on the GMC, most of which was spent dealing with drunken Irish doctors. The difference between an Irishman and an Englishman is that when an Englishman totters out of the Café Royale and a policeman says to him 'Ave a good evening, Governor, let me take care of your keys and get you a taxi.' The Englishman duly does so and collects his car next day. The Irishman in the same situation retorts – 'Accusing me of being bloody well drunk, are you?' and then knocks the policeman down for good measure.

At one stage he guided me towards a large window.

There, that is the graveyard; so we know exactly where we are going, we have some vague idea whence we came – it is the in-between that is irritating, but there is little we can do about it. There is no point in dwelling on the past, nothing that is past can be altered, so why think about it? Ten o'clock this morning is gone irretrievably, so therefore, I never dwell on the past.

Dom Peter Flood died on 16 December 1978, at the age of eighty.

PART TWO

The Corruption of Privilege

Medical Education

I BECAME FRIENDLY in the 1970s with Michael O'Donnell, the flamboyant editor of the avidly read *World Medicine*. I wrote a number of pieces, many anonymously, for this remarkable journal that flowered briefly from 1966 to 1982. In *World Medicine* the infamously outspoken editor stimulated debate on areas of the medical establishment – most notably the General Medical Council – that deemed themselves above and beyond comment, not to mention censure. Michael probably did more for the health of medicine in the UK in this period than any of the long-established journals, such as the *British Medical Journal* and *The Lancet*, which were by tradition very conservative in tone and expression. He encouraged writers, such as me, to question the traditions and established tenants of medical practice. In the essay 'Six Years Shalt Thou Labour'[1] written in 1973 I question the need for such a six-year apprenticeship in medicine. In the essay 'History, Diagnosis and *then* Examination'[2] I challenge the traditional procedure of taking a history and examining the patient before arriving at a diagnosis. I am even more convinced today of the truth in the statement 'that if for the rest of my medical days I was to be given the choice of either taking a history or examining the patient, I would without hesitation settle for the former option'.

'Towards Being a Scientific Doctor and the Dangers of the Dublin Disease'[3] written in 1982 is a plea for clinical research to be given a place under the sun and a recognition of the temptation for the doctor with academic ability to succumb to the 'babble of the market', sublimating the call for enquiry and research in the face of the fiscal rewards of private practice. This I dubbed 'The Dublin Disease', an affliction that may be more rampant in the city the name of which it bears but which is, in fact, endemic in university teaching hospitals worldwide.

The first medical institute to influence my career was the Royal College of Surgeons in Ireland, where both my parents had graduated in medicine, and which afforded me a welcome escape from Castleknock College, which once fled was never revisited. My premature exit from this establishment was achieved through my espousing my father's advice that dentistry was a career to my liking, medicine then being considered over-crowded – 'thirteen-to-the-dozen' was a popular phrase – whereas dentists were prospering. The alternative to spending another year at school was to enter 'MacDowall's grind' in York Street so as to sit the matriculation or entrance examination to the College rather than wait another year at school to sit the Leaving Certificate. Success in this endeavour enabled me to enter the College as a dental student in September 1957.

In the 1960s medical and dental students sat the same examinations for the first three years (known as the pre-clinical years) before parting company – the former to spend the next three years attached to teaching hospitals and the latter destined to imprisonment in the Dental Hospital on Lincoln Place. Here I spent three months in a state of indolence and apathy. The zero achieved in my first examination, Dental Metallurgy, was a disappointment to me. I had expected the examiner to award my answer to the question, 'Discuss the uses of wire in dentistry' with at least a mark or two for iconoclastic originality. Having recently re-wired the complex system of bells that extended from room to room in the family home I was an authority on this topic, and my answer to the use of wire in dentistry ran to some three pages. One of these was devoted to a drawing of a Georgian doorway on Merrion Square, clearly depicted as being the portal of entry to the dentist, with the doorbell as the focal point from which wires emanated to a transformer faithfully carrying the vital impulses to the nidus of fulfilment – the bell, with its little clapper deep within the bowels of the sanctum, alerting the buxom blonde receptionist that a patient was nigh, and without which the product of six years training would be denied sustenance – surely the greatest use for wire in the profession! Following this result even my father had to admit that dentistry was not my avocation and so after three months adrift of my colleagues I turned to medicine, readjusted my sights and spent the next three happy years as a clinical clerk 'walking the wards' of the Richmond Hospital. Perhaps I was beginning to question the rigidity of establishment medicine?

I qualified as a doctor in June 1963, but my involvement with RCSI continued first as a research fellow, later as clinical teacher, acting professor of pharmacology and therapeutics (from July 1973 to October 1975), professor of cardiovascular medicine (from November 1991 to April 2001), professor of cardiovascular pharmacology (from April 2001 to December 2004), and editor of the college journal on two occasions (from 1973 to 1977 and from 1987 to 1993).

My affection for the College of Surgeons was considerable and is probably best discerned through the many essays and books I wrote or edited relating to the College and its teaching hospitals.

My personal favourite has to be *A Portrait of Irish Medicine*,[4] which was published to mark the bicentenary of the Royal College of Surgeons in Ireland in 1984. In this book Anne Crookshank and I set out to portray the progress and development of Irish medicine through painting, engraving, sculpture, stained glass photography and architecture. Together we visited museums, galleries, medical institutions, churches, cathedrals and private collections throughout Ireland. What a pleasure it was for me to have such a wonderfully knowledgeable and delightfully eccentric companion. Many of the works we chose to reproduce in *A Portrait* are of considerable artistic interest; some are largely unknown and many had never been reproduced before. A deluxe edition of *A Portrait* in full leather with the spine depicting the barber's pole – an emblem of surgery to this day – is now much sought after by book collectors.[5]

The essay 'What is a Professor?' owes its existence to an unusual event that took place in Dublin in 1979.[6] I would not have written on the issue were it not for an attempt by a senior colleague to prevent me expressing my views on the subject. As is explained in the essay, a pharmaceutical company had decided to endow two chairs in cardiology in one of Dublin's universities and to mark the occasion a lavish jamboree was arranged in the newly opened, opulent Berkeley Court Hotel. Unfortunately inclement weather at Heathrow Airport delayed the arrival of a contingent of dignitaries from the cardiological establishment in Britain, with the result that the welcoming gathering, drawn from the highest reaches of the profession in Ireland, imbibed rather more than might have been judicious even for such an occasion. When eventually all were seated for dinner it became apparent to Walter Somerville, the then editor of the *British Heart Journal*,[7] that the state of inebriation that greeted the sober contingent from London was not confined to the guests; one waiter dispensed soup liberally on the carpet as he pirouetted from table to table. Walter, in an act of customary kindness, hastily wrote on the back of the place card bearing his name, 'My dear fellow, you have had a little too much to drink and would be well advised to go home.' Without reading the card the waiter waddled off to another table and duly delivered the message to a distinguished London professor who was not renowned for intemperance or humour.

In the course of this bacchanalian evening I expressed my reservations about endowed chairs, stating that it was a travesty to have endowed two chairs in one university and that it demeaned the title, adding that it was a subject deserving of debate. I would probably not have given the matter another thought were it not for the fact that I was phoned early the following morning by a senior colleague who advised me that if I had thoughts on airing the subject in print I would be well advised to desist from doing so.

Reading this essay again from a distance of many years I could hardly have anticipated that I would add substance to the concluding prediction that 'Dublin would soon earn a reputation similar to that which it once had as a city of "dreadful knights" of now being one of "dismal professors".' After all, I have held no fewer than three chairs and declined a fourth. Shortly after being appointed to my first chair I told Samuel Beckett at one of our meetings in Paris that he could now call me 'Professor'. He replied that this was 'wonderful' and congratulated me warmly. I felt obliged however to declare that my chair was only a personal one and being asked to expound I went on to explain that a personal chair was in recognition of scientific achievement and that it did not carry administrative or teaching duties, that in fact you carried on just as before except that the proletariat might feel more obliged to tip the cap, as it were. 'Well, Eoin,' he said, 'sounds more like a stool than a chair,' and warming to the analogy went on, 'but to be sure stools are much more useful than chairs, especially in bars where they allow the arse to be propped in propinquity to the elbow, the one balanced nicely in concert with the other so as to clutch the pint twixt counter and gob.'

Six Years Shalt Thou Labour ... , 1979

'WHAT'S THAT CALLED?' said my son, pointing to a tendon in his foot, as I consoled him after he had twisted his ankle.

'I'm afraid I don't know,' I replied unthinkingly.

'But I thought you were a doctor,' said he, in some amazement.

In fact, so did I.

My son's concept of a doctor as an individual capable of answering any question relating to the body is perfectly understandable; he is, after all, a 'lay boy', and moreover is only seven. When, however, medical men of mature years, who also happen to be the ones who structure medical school curricula, arrange for the trainee doctor to be packed full of nonsense during six long years, so that he may subsequently, at least in theory, approach my son's ideal of omnipotent knowledge, should we not question their suitability for the educational task at hand? You see, I, of all people, should have been able to give my son the correct answer to his question. I began my medical career in dentistry, and after two years of anatomy instruction, it was indeed a foolish dental student who did not know every anatomical detail of the foot, the likelihood being that in the examination his knowledge would be tested in this extremity rather than (as would seem more appropriate to any reasonable individual) on the anatomical peculiarities of the skull. It can be said with some truth that times have changed, but have they changed all that much? We continue to put our medical students through six long years of apprenticeship and, if anything, today's curriculum contains more irrelevant detail than did mine. Moreover, the student is under the constant pressure of continuous assessment with less time for recreation, relaxation, and development of the whole man so essential to the development of a good doctor. Doctors are expensive to produce but they are needed, if not here, elsewhere in the world. We are endeavouring to cut back on the student intake so as to reduce the doctor output. There is, in my view, no reason why we cannot train in four years doctors every bit as competent as those passing out of medical schools today after six long years.

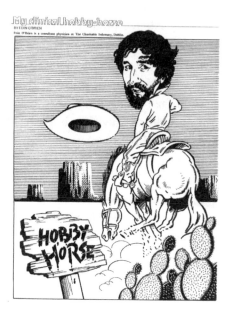

Cartoon of the author from World Medicine, *1979.*

Looking back on my medical student days, there is only one period that now seems important to me, and that is the time I spent (much of it in residence) as a clinical clerk in the Richmond Hospital. I recall those happy times vividly. There on the wards by the bedside, in the casualty and out-patients and in the theatre, was the doctor in me formed. The residency period should be increased rather than contracted (as is the practice in some schools) and the student should be freed from lectures and other commitments so that he can, by becoming a member of the team to which he is attached, absorb medicine at first hand. (The same applies to his apprenticeship in general practice, a welcome concept in training, which was not accepted when I was a student.) Presumably the trainee pilot spends much of his time in the cockpit, as does a musician at the piano, but medical students are actually being taken further and further away from the bedside and practical training.

I can scarcely remember anything from the physics and chemistry that were crammed into me during the pre-med year; I suppose I could answer a few very general questions on these subjects, but I suspect that I had thrown out most of this year's toil by the time I started to walk the wards. Biology did have some relevance, and a study of the amoeba, dogfish, and frog did at least introduce one to the methodology later to be applied to the human species. The standard of science has improved in our schools, and I cannot see any valid argument for retaining pre-med, which saves us our first year.

Was not the division of medical education into pre-clinical and clinical years most unfortunate? On the one side is a group of more or less full-time teachers who rarely, if ever, have any contact with patients, and on the other are the part-time hospital teachers who rarely if ever communicate with their pre-clinical colleagues. Each side stagnating in apathetic isolation gives but little thought to what is best for the doctor in the making. Only recently have medical educators questioned the validity of this arbitrary division, and it seems to me sound sense to integrate, for example, the teaching of anatomy with that of radiology and surgery. And while talking of anatomy, it is with the greatest resentment that I look back on two years spent in memorizing list after list of useless facts to satisfy examiners in a minor specialty, which had somehow over the ages acquired educational status out of all proportion to its worth. Even had I become a surgeon, the anatomical knowledge acquired in my student days would have been discarded before I embarked on specialist training, the purpose of which would be to teach me the whole subject once again in greater depth. I do not know if there still exists the divide between physiology and applied physiology but, if such does exist, I for one fail to see the wisdom in this dichotomy. Should not all subjects be *applied* to illness, which is after all what we are setting out to alleviate, and does any subject better lend itself to this than physiology? Which brings me back to this question of integration of disciplines. The student should be brought into contact with the patient as soon as possible, and by that I mean in his first year at medical school. How much time is wasted in attempting to apply, for example, physiological and pathological concepts to illnesses, which are but distant myths?

Another aspect of this retrospective analysis seems to be, if anything, a greater problem today than when I was a student, and that is the 'empire building' mania, which is the result of each professorial department being given almost total autonomy in its development. So it happens that a discipline of relatively minor importance may, by virtue of the energies of its seemingly well-motivated professor, demand from the students an inordinate lecture attendance, and impose upon them examinations of an exemplary standard. Failure to satisfy the examiners in these minor subjects may well have the same disastrous consequences for the student as if he had failed one of the major disciplines. It is difficult to see how this problem can be resolved, but every medical school must view critically any proposed expansion of the curriculum, and ensure that a delicate balance is maintained between subjects of major and minor importance – the balance not being constant, but changing as development may modify society's requirements from its doctors. Careful planning and judicious allocation of time to each subject according to its importance, the integration of teaching between disciplines where indicated, and the avoidance of repetition in the curriculum, could save another year.

Further savings might be possible if we could change our attitude to knowledge, which for the most part we equate with our ability to memorize, an important but exaggerated aspect of medical education, which is clearly demonstrated in our dedication to the MCQ examination. I remember a fellow student who, alas, did not survive much beyond the first half; he was a little older than most of us, and had an intelligent disregard for the medical curriculum. He studied, but not too often, preferring to indulge himself in Wagner, Racine, and an occasional woman, not necessarily in that order, of course. What studies he did were directed towards spotting the questions most likely to arise in the examination and towards this end he attended diligently the last lectures of the term. With the occult assistance of an out-of-work gypsy fortune-teller whose professional lack of success with the crystal ball, he assured us, was but a reflection on her utter devotion to more earthy matters (the likes of which the rest of us but dreamed of) he had remarkable success in predicting the papers. Never wishing to tax his mind unduly, he would appear at the examination wearing a greatcoat (ultimately to be his downfall on a sweltering June day) which was, in effect, an ingenious contraption in the substance of which were secreted away the answers to the selected questions.

A great believer in the potential of the dawning electronic age, he had for many months earned the sympathy of his teachers by wearing a hearing aid through which he hoped to have transmitted information that would permit him to pass with ease not only the papers, but also the viva. Why is it necessary for the student to carry around in his small cerebrum the contents of a library? He must, of course, be capable of retaining basic knowledge on some of the many topics that constitute medicine, but is it not more important that he should know how to find knowledge than that he should retain it indefinitely, which, we would all admit, is quite impossible? It would be better to spend more time in showing the student how to find information and, having found it, how to assess it critically – some of our examinations could be well directed towards this end. In practice is it not experience (a very different phenomenon from mere learning) that permits us to cope with most medical problems? And, when we do come up against the occasional rarity, do we not seek help from the literature or a specialist colleague?

A firm, wise, and diplomatic director (I nearly said dictator) of medical education, be he called dean or whatever, could, if given a free hand in readjusting the balance of power among the different disciplines, not only shorten the medical course to four years without lowering the present standards, but he could also return to medical students some of the recreational time that was their right until recently, so that they might develop with a healthier outlook on life. Let us end with the words of William Stokes who advocated a liberal education for medical students: 'Let us emancipate the student, and give him time and opportunity for the cultivation of his mind, so that in his pupilage he be not a puppet in the hands of others, but rather a self-relying and reflecting being.'

History, Diagnosis and then Examination, 1979

IN THE COURSE of a year's teaching to students, during which time much is said, only one exhortation is worthy of recall. To the junior students, arriving fresh from three years' deprivation in the preclinical wilderness, I stress and attempt to illustrate that the patient's history is much more important in reaching a diagnosis than will be the information gleaned from physical examination. I say, quite truthfully, that if for the rest of my medical days I were to be given the choice of either taking a history or examining the patient, I would without hesitation settle for the former option. I speak, of course, for my own speciality of cardiology, but perhaps the situation is not all that different in other disciplines – more of that later. I urge them to leave that talisman of medical approbation in the hip pocket, where a discreet showing of the earpieces will serve them far better in social advancement than in clinical achievement.

When I come to teach the final-year students I realize that the message of three years earlier has been forgotten or suppressed in the course of later training. Having stressed once more the importance of devoting the major part of clinical assessment to the history, I advise them to pause after taking the history, to make a differential diagnosis, and then to examine the patient selectively.

Some students regard this approach as a little short of fair play. Unfortunately they come to finals believing in the concept of a 'complete physical', something that none of their teachers have attempted to do since qualifying.

A careful history and relevant examination will permit a diagnosis, or a few differential diagnoses (as distinct from an endless list of 'problems') in almost every patient, and this being so, investigations if indicated at all, need be few. Students must learn that there is no such thing as a 'routine investigation'; that all investigations must be ordered only after careful thought; that all investigations cause the patient discomfort and that investigations are very costly. (Hospitals should publish regularly a list of the costs of investigations for the education of doctors, nurses and students.)

Some time ago, writing in *World Medicine*,[8] I earned the opprobrium of a geriatrician for decrying excessive investigation, particularly in the elderly, and I concluded that 'most clinicians know the answer at the end of a thorough history and clinical examination; in fact, usually make the diagnosis at the end of the history'. Maurice Pappworth, not one to mince his words, wrote in my defence that 'it is usually the clinicians of poor calibre who attempt to justify the multiplicity of their investigations on the grounds of thoroughness, or fear of missing something or playing for time … merely because the facilities are available for a particular test is not a sensible reason for ordering it'.

The sceptic might dismiss what has gone above as anecdotal conjecture were it not for an interesting and valuable article by Gerald Sandler in the *British Medical Journal* entitled 'Costs of Unnecessary Tests'.[9] The diagnoses in 630 patients referred to a medical outpatients department were carefully analyzed. The accuracy of diagnosis made by the general practitioner, the junior hospital staff and the consultant was assessed, and then the influence of the history, the examination and investigations on both diagnosis and management was studied.

The history provided the diagnosis in two-thirds of patients, and it also decided management in nearly half of all patients. In patients presenting with chest pain, 90 per cent can be diagnosed from the history alone. The examination, on the other hand, affected diagnosis and management in only 17 per cent of cases.

Examination gave the least help in gastrointestinal disease and was of most help in respiratory disease, and less so in cardiovascular disease where its main importance was in the diagnosis of hypertension and valvular heart disease.

But what of investigations? So-called 'routine' blood count, erythrocyte sedimentation rate, blood urea and serum electrolyte estimations were of diagnostic help in only 1 per cent of patients. Urine examination, blood sugar estimation, chest X-rays and ECGs were of little help in a 'routine' capacity, but if these are regarded as a special investigation in patients with diabetes, respiratory and cardiovascular disease, understandably their value is greater. Of the special investigations, the most useful were barium studies and cholecystograms in deciding the diagnosis of alimentary problems. Likewise, thyroid function tests and glucose tolerance tests were helpful in endocrine disease.

The annual saving to the National Health Service in Britain if no routine tests were done would be around £3.5 million and, as the author points out, 'the corresponding loss of help in diagnosis and management would be negligible'.

This fiscal conclusion will, of course, be of interest to the administrators, who must by now know that bureaucratic dissipation of finance in the health services is matched only by the thoughtless extravagance of the medical profession. But Doctor Sandler has another important message – this one for teachers of medical students. He points out that conventional training is based on the concept that only after a history and examination can a diagnosis be considered. On the basis of his study he advocates that 'the traditional case presentation of history and examination followed by differential diagnosis should be changed to history, diagnosis and *relevant* examination findings'. It is time for an iconoclastic revision of our clinical teaching methods.

The Dangers of the Dublin Disease, 1982

ONE OF OUR saner medical philosophers, Richard Asher, said, 'The whole art of medicine depends on the stimuli that enter the mind of the physician (or that structure corresponding to a mind in the surgeon), the processes that goes on in that mind, and the material produced by that mind, as a result.' [10]

It is helpful in considering the research doctor to concentrate on these three fundamental processes. Greatness, whether applied to the individual or to major advance is dependent on these associated functions.

Under the first of Asher's premises – that which enters the mind – we must direct our attention to what we teach the research doctor and how we train him. Do we teach our doctors research technique? The answer in general terms has to be that we do not for the very simple reason that with a few exceptions, we are not capable of teaching research technique, being ourselves untutored in scientific method. Clinicians must not react to this criticism by putting up the inevitable defence: 'I am a service doctor; that is what I was trained for and that is what I am good at.' Fair comment but the addendum that 'these research allecadoos couldn't tell a tonsil from a thyroid' furthers the case not at all. If clinicians are not themselves inclined towards research, they must not deny the species space in which to ripen. They must appreciate their worth. Let the clinical doctor not forget that his knowledge and ability to practice his art is dependent on the research of his predecessors. There is another reason why students and graduates should be knowledgeable about research technique and scientific method, and that is so that they can appreciate and judge critically the ever-expanding volume of scientific work in medicine.

So much for teaching; of even greater importance in considering that which enters the mind of the scientific doctor is the training with which he is provided. There are two very important defects in our system. Firstly, Ireland can only provide a very limited training for the scientifically minded doctor. However, as the country's academic stature grows – and it is developing – this deficiency can be overcome by placing promising graduates in centres of excellence abroad.

The second fault in the system is not so easily overcome. If it is accepted that a proportion of doctors should be trained to become research workers, there must be room for them in the career structure. At present the hospital and academic career structures are such that extraordinarily few doctors can find secure tenure in full-time academic scientific work. This is to the detriment of the profession: where are the readers and lecturers with consultant status? Not very long ago the plea might have been – where are the full-time professors?

Ireland is very much behind the times in academic development. Professor Leslie Witts in his Harveian Oration given over a decade ago estimated that apart from professors, a professorial unit to be effective needed also: 'at least two senior assistants, and a non-medical graduate with security of tenure, in addition to two or three junior assistants who will maintain the infusion of new blood and provide the next cohort of trained workers'.[11] He went on, 'There will also be a number of attached workers on research grants of one kind or another, many of them working for a higher degree.' Leslie Wilts was outlining the professorial unit, as it existed in Britain, and in many other European countries. There is a lack of will in the profession here to influence government towards accepting the need for an alteration in the career structuring of academic posts to provide the occupant with consultant status. The fault rests with the profession and not with the government, which will respond only when pressure is applied.

Let us assume that the mind of our scientific doctor has been prepared by exposure to knowledge and experience during the training period. This, at least, fulfils Pasteur's aphorism that 'Fortune favours the prepared mind.' But the scientifically minded doctor is going to need more than a mind prepared by crude medical or scientific knowledge. His mind must be, above all, capable of discerning – or as Sir William Hale White once remarked, 'It has been truly said that for one person who can see, fifty can think.' It is the quality of being able to see that will make the research worker excel. This gift can be cultivated by a broad knowledge of scientific endeavour, and by an appreciation of other disciplines and of the humanities. No mind should be constrained within the straitjacket of its own discipline, or it will wither in its own sterility. The scientific doctor should have other characteristics as well – his personality should be vibrant and receptive; his character generous and above the petty jealousies that so bedevil the progress of lesser men; above all he must have integrity and a sincere commitment to pursuing the goal of achievement through research. The researcher must not take his status for granted if he or she is fortunate enough to be granted full-time academic status, the luxury of a more leisurely existence must not be snatched as an opportunity to further some other gainful sideline; it is for the development of his intellect, and for the enrichment of the minds of those around him.

If clinicians view academe with some scepticism it is because they can point their fingers at many full-time academics and ask in vain for the produce of their scientific endeavour. It is difficult for academic authorities to establish a means of accountability within their departments when in effect the government of the institute is to a large extent in the hands of the heads of these departments. But accountability there must be, and it is long overdue in Ireland.

Now let us assume that our young doctor has been prepared adequately for the role of a research worker, and let us assume that the produce of his young mind is promising and that he is casting his eye towards Dublin as the place in which he would like to work and live. There is one very important step to be taken – he or she must vaccinate his or her mind against the Dublin Disease.

This syndrome has not hitherto been described and this journal is therefore privileged in being the first to publish the results of a study conducted over a twenty-year period. The scientific and statistical methods are impeccable and details are available on request from the author.

The Dublin Disease has been so named, not because it is confined to this metropolis, but because the effects of the illness have been most devastating in the environs of Anna Livia. The condition exists to be sure in other Irish cities – Cork and Galway being notable examples and epidemics have been known to occur in America. It is however, rare in virulent form in Great Britain. Originally it was thought to be confined to the male sex and never to occur before thirty-five years of age. Both these assumptions are now known to be incorrect. It is, however, unique in being confined, as presently described, to the medical profession. A typical case report will serve to illustrate the condition, though there are fifty cases in this study spreading over three generations.

The young doctor, usually male, graduates with honours in a number of subjects and proceeds to a professorial non-consultant hospital appointment. During this period he is ambitious, idealistic, to the left of centre in politics, well-behaved, occasionally promiscuous and given betimes to bouts of bacchanalian debauchery, during which he vents his spleen on the medical system in Dublin, on his boss in particular, and in moments of great excess to his boss in person. A remarkable feature is his ability to survive such incidents. He is vehement in his disapproval of private practice although the acquirement of a mate seems to weaken his stance on this principle. He willingly makes personal and family sacrifices in the further-ance of his career and is successful in obtaining coveted positions abroad. Here he endears himself to all with whom he comes in contact. He acquires specialist research training and publishes prolifically in the international journals. He is invited home to promote his work, and his image, and ultimately he applies for and succeeds in obtaining a consultant appointment in a teaching hospital. It is now that the first signs of the Dublin Disease become manifest. The symptoms are insidious at first. He asks the management committee for space, a secretary and some equipment – modest requirements compared to what he has been accus-tomed to. His requests are usually ignored and sometimes refused out of hand. He begins to complain. He is seen to throw up his arms in characteristic gesture when talking to his younger colleagues, and he begins to view his older colleagues with suspicion. When intemperate his choler knows no bounds, and his language is not at all scientific.

A small notice appears in the social and personal column of *The Irish Times* stating that he has taken rooms. The Department of Health has long recognized the syndrome, and is indeed culpable in masking its symptoms by palliative medi-cine. The Board of Management having held out for a prescribed length of time eventually purchase for their new arrival an expensive Japanese diagnostiscope in the use of which he has excelled abroad and his colleagues begin to refer patients to him. The hospital management notices with complacent relief that he is no longer making a nuisance of himself phoning and writing for space and equipment. His medical colleagues observe that he is generally of a more contented mien, a little more corpulent in stature, dressed very nattily, and moving about the city on a smooth set of wheels. They are glad to see that he is settling in.

At parties he is now heard to utter that research in this country is pointless, we are too small, even if we had the funding we wouldn't have the numbers. Doctors from Dublin visiting his centre of training abroad are asked by his disappointed mentors: 'Whatever happened to O'Nobel – he never seems to publish and he did show such promise.' How could they know that he has succumbed to the Dublin Disease? This disease is common, its consequences tragic for Irish medicine and its cure rests not with the individuals afflicted but with the academic and governmental institutes of the country. If we wish to protect our bright young doctors from what Gogarty once called the 'babble of the market', we must then recompense them adequately for their labours in academe. It is pointless to criticize anyone for seeking in private practice a reward that is vastly greater than anything that might be obtained in the public or academic sector. Doctors, in common with the rest of mankind, can resist anything except temptation.

Now let us assume that stages one and two of Asher's dictates have been met – namely that what has gone into the mind of the young scientist has been influenced judiciously and that his mind has been intelligent enough to assimilate that knowledge, and to come up with an observation or discovery of note. One might then say – well what more is there to it – now all he or she has to do is spew out the results at an international meeting, and subsequently in a prestigious journal, and then the individual and his institute can sit back and wait for glory. It is not so simple – Asher's third concern about the material produced by the mind must be heeded.

Graduates are rarely instructed in the art of communication. This inability to communicate is apparent at an early stage. It can be detected in the undergraduate examination essays – how awful they are, and the awful practice continues unabated into the postgraduate sphere. What a pity that the examinee cannot be subjected to the misery that is the lot of the examiner. How much he would modify his technique. Let students picture their favourite – or better still their not so favourite – examiner, lolling in his garden on a beautiful Sunday afternoon in spring. The sun, the birds, the fragrance of the flowers, the warmth, and perhaps a little vintage burgundy assail the senses, and induce a torpor that sets a troubled soul at ease. In short the sort of day in which, to quote Samuel Beckett, it is difficult to keep God out of one's thoughts. But out he must go for there on the table are 100 essay questions awaiting correction for Monday morning. I received during my undergraduate training in this College two salutary lessons – both in the art of communication, and both from one man – the kindly and enigmatic professor of physiology, Frank Kane. He greatly disliked the habit of constant note taking during his lectures, but students being students would not heed the advice of this, in their opinion, eccentric little man. One day in the midst of a lecture on Starling's Law, he went on: 'The force of contraction of the heart muscle made the rats die and the stench was awful.' He then stopped his talk and asked a Trinidadian beauty to read her notes, which, like so many others in the class, contained his exact words.

Kane's other lesson to me was to be of greater importance than all the knowledge I so readily learned ultimately to forget. It was his policy to set for us a Christmas exam after which he would take us aside individually and discuss – not so much the results, which were usually dismal, but our method of presenting our very meagre store of knowledge. I recall that his comments to me went something like this: 'You have what I might call a quaint knowledge of physiology, and a commendable talent for improvisation that may be a distinct advantage, but if you were to blend this characteristic with an intelligent technique, who knows you might yet qualify.' He advised me to have compassion for the unfortunate examiner, to pity his terrible plight, to remember that he might be ageing and that his sight might be failing and that it was a foolish student who expected him to read through pages of nonsense seeking the rare jewel of knowledge therein. He advised me to make his task easy by structuring my answer. Ever since I have done essay questions according to his format: 'I propose to answer the question under the following headings 1, 2, 3.' 'You see,' he said, 'in this way the examiner doesn't have to read all the nonsense you write, he just marks you for the knowledge you have and subtracts for that which you obviously don't possess.'

How is it that we neglect to place the subject of communication on our curriculum? As a profession we are so dependent on it. We write an awful lot of letters, most of them awful. We need to be able to present ourselves to our peers, and yet we come out of medical school incapable of writing a curriculum vitae. When it comes to presenting the results of our research work on the stage or in a journal the effect is very often pathetic.

If money is to be invested in producing scientific workers they must be capable of communicating their observations. This is not easy. There are many excellent books on the subject but these are read only by those already competent. There have been postgraduate courses but again these usually preach to the converted. There is a very real place for instruction in the art of communication at undergraduate level. At least it should be possible to make the student aware of the limitations of communication, and to instruct him how to present his knowledge be it for an exam, a talk, a publication or simply for a curriculum vitae on which his advancement is so dependent.

Two decades ago this College was a school that merely produced doctors – doctors who were competent, very competent – in the practice of medicine. It was not and did not pride itself on being an academic institute in the generally accepted meaning of that term. Few of its graduates aspired to academic status. Indeed few could do so. The university doors were barred to licentiates who were not eligible for postgraduate degrees. Indeed special permission had to be sought to sit for membership examinations of the Royal Colleges. The academic departments were run on a part-time basis to provide undergraduate education with little thought being given to postgraduate development.

The graduates then fitted nicely into Shaw's scheme of things. 'As a matter of fact,' that wise Irishman said, 'the rank and file of doctors are no more scientific than their tailors; or, if you prefer to put it the reverse way their tailors are no less scientific than they.' And he doesn't stop there. 'It does happen exceptionally that a practising doctor makes a contribution to science; but it happens much oftener that he draws disastrous conclusions from his clinical experience because he has no conception of scientific method, and believes, like any rustic, that the handling of evidence and statistics needs no expertness.' What wisdom there is in this statement!

Four significant events have changed the course of the College. The new building showed the Higher Education Authority and others that there was still life in the old girl and much credit must go to Harry O'Flanagan for this achievement. Next came a demand from the graduates who sought the same opportunities as graduates of other medical schools. They sought entrance to academe and the College wisely read the signs and there followed what I shall call the marriage with University College Dublin, which now grants to our progeny respectability and acceptance in academic society. Now the College has begun to fund research, and this is a very significant step forward.

The bodybuilding phase is over and an era of intellectual development is now mandatory. The College may, in fact, be in a unique and privileged position in which to advance medical research and achievement in this country. Unilateral expansion of the medical faculties of our universities would not be permitted to any significant degree by other disciplines that would see their own development as being just as important as that of medicine. The College has no such restraints on development. However, if it is to become a centre of excellence – and that is, I hope, what all would wish for it – it has to realize that the cost is going to be considerably greater than that of erecting buildings, and the planning far more complex and critical. It is, therefore, imperative that it deploys its funds wisely. A centre of excellence requires, first and foremost, people of excellence. The College must appoint those who have shown through their labours their academic worth, and their ability to achieve excellence. Now if the College is going to attract these men and women, it must establish an environment in which excellence can thrive. Francis Wood wrote in 1967: 'I tried to make a place where the finest, most intelligent young gentlemen would want to come to work and stay … Anything that contributes to this purpose is good; anything that interferes with it is bad, and anything that does not affect it is unimportant.' The College could do well to adopt these sentiments.

In their present state, the major departments of the College are for the greater part deplorable in academic terms; and these must be developed without delay. The College must not permit the proliferation of undergraduate professorial departments until the major departments are fully developed, nor should it merely increase the numbers of its academic staff by, for example, incorporating other institutes under its academic umbrella. The people needed must be sought for carefully to fulfil the contingencies of a well-planned academic programme. The College must avoid haphazard and seemingly convenient expediencies, which may be to its long-term detriment.

The first step is to provide the major departments with – in addition to whole-time professors – readers, senior lecturers, and research fellows, many of whom will have to be given security of tenure, which calls for some re-thinking in the relationship between the academics and hospital consultants. And then there has to be money for research itself. These are costly ambitions but this institute has shown itself more than capable of overcoming what seemed at one time to be insurmountable odds. If it now turns its talents and ingenuity towards its intellectual development it can and will become a relevant force in our science of healing the sick.

What is a Professor?, 1979

WHAT IS A professor? The question appears deceptively simple yet the answer is difficult to provide. Fearing that my interpretation of the title was becoming outmoded, I sat down to think and ultimately to write.

Recourse to the Oxford Dictionary did little to resolve matters. A chair is 'a seat of authority, state, or dignity... from which a professor or other authorised teacher delivers his lectures' and a professor is 'a public teacher, or instructor of the highest rank in a specific faculty or branch of learning'. There were of course many other uses of the terms, and although attracted by the description of a chair as 'an attribute of old age, when rest is the natural condition', I discarded the dictionary as a source of inspiration or further information.

There can be little doubt about the general public's assessment of a professor. The title is regarded as a rank of excellence, which indeed it should be. After all, if the academic institute bestows upon one of its members its highest rank, is it not quite reasonable to assume that this is a collective tribute to wisdom? But the public interpretation of the term, although relevant, is not as important as our own concept of the professorial role.

Most of our chairs have been established by the academic institutes to which they belong, but occasionally an institute sees fit to bestow a personal chair upon one of its members as a tribute for outstanding work and achievement in one of the specialities.

Established chairs are usually filled by open competition, and are generally financed by the institute either wholly or as a proportion of total salary. In recent years and rather belatedly our universities are appointing whole-time professors and private practice is limited, with income over a certain level being returned to the institute. In the major specialities such as medicine and surgery it is not uncommon to have two professors rotate the chairmanship of the department between them at fixed intervals. This practice is good but might be taken a little further. Why not limit tenure of office to ten or fifteen years? This would encourage a total commitment to academic development during the occupant's most productive years and on completion of office he could be given the title of emeritus professor. If there are to be two or more professors in one discipline they should be chosen for individual qualities that would ensure the rational development of a productive department. For example, one might be appointed for his research abilities, and another for his teaching or administrative skills.

Obviously it is desirable that chairs in the major disciplines should be occupied by full-time professors and it should go without saying that those appointed to established chairs should have an impressive academic record. They should be committed to the ideal of academic development, so that their fulfilment would come from this, and they should not, as Gogarty once said speaking in another vein, be distracted by the 'babble of the market'. This, of course, means that universities must ensure that their full-time professors are paid a realistic wage, bearing in mind that in most specialities the private sector will be a constant temptation to even the most stoic academic.

The practice of appointing associate or assistant professors can, in my view, only lead to dissatisfaction, and there must ultimately be ill feeling if, as happens, the incumbent regards the chair as his by right. It would be far better if our academic departments were properly staffed with readers and lecturers than bolstered with very part-time assistant professors. Our medical schools do not appear to realize that well structured professorial departments have been in existence and have been operating productively over many years in most other countries. In his Harvian Oration in 1971, Leslie Witts estimated that in Great Britain 'the average medical professorial unit might be presumed to consist of eight people paid by the university and a similar number of attached workers'. Though our departments are improving, they are doing so at a tortuously slow pace. A major fault with our established chairs is a total lack of accountability for performance. It is not enough anymore to train medical students so that they become reasonably competent doctors. The professor of any department is responsible for this to be sure, but he must also see that his department as well as being a seat of learning is an area of active research and scientific enquiry. To do this he has to develop his department, acquire and direct his staff, and the fruits of his efforts are to be judged by the calibre of his scientific communications and publications. It should be the practice of all medical teaching institutes to produce an annual report clearly depicting the undergraduate and postgraduate activities of each department and, perhaps more important, a list of published work, the worth of which will be readily apparent.

So much for established chairs, but what of personal chairs? Is it not high time that we took a close look at this means of approbation, which, if misused, could do a grave disservice to our academic standards? As I see it, an institute may rarely – very rarely – see fit to honour a member whose contribution to his discipline has been significant and outstanding. Provided such an individual exists, the means of endowing his chair is probably not very relevant, and it would matter little whether the money came from the university or from industry. Great would be the threat to the integrity of our academic standards if, for example, the pharmaceutical industry by merely providing money was permitted to endow chairs in a particular speciality, or for an individual of its choosing.

Recently, a pharmaceutical company endowed no less than two chairs in cardiology in one university. It would seem to me quite reasonable, desirable and indeed deserving that there should be one endowed chair of cardiology in this country, but to create two chairs in a small speciality, both in Dublin and both in the same university, makes a farce of the whole professorial concept and raises some ethical considerations as well. The die is now apparently cast, the university has given its approval, and the chairs will be filled shortly. There might seem then to be little point in running the risk of opprobrium by writing frankly about this issue, but my reason for doing so is that I see a most undesirable precedent being established. If it becomes common practice for endowed chairs to be established in this manner in the specialities, Dublin would soon earn a reputation similar to that which it once had as a city of 'dreadful knights', now being one of 'dismal professors'.

The Medical Establishment

RECENTLY I EXPRESSED to my friend Paddy MacEntee my concern that I was being brought into conflict with the establishment of my profession at a time in my life when such relationships should be tranquil rather than confrontational. How was it, I asked him, that in the course of one year I should have to challenge the Royal College of Surgeons (an institution for which I had both affection and respect and which I had served for so long) for its stance in Bahrain, and that I found it necessary for the same reason to resign my fellowship of the Royal College of Physicians? Paddy, having pondered briefly, put my dilemma succinctly into context in his inimitable way: 'Eoin, you are merely sensing what perhaps you did not have the time, or the wisdom, to heed hithertofore – *the corruption of privilege.*'

How right he was. Institutions, be they medical, legal, political or religious, are privileged by virtue of the influence they wield in society, but they are further privileged in that they control the fate of their practitioners, who must aspire to impress their masters and to whom it is made very clear that to transgress can be foolhardy in the extreme. Paddy was also correct in sensing that I had not previously had the time (nor perhaps the courage) to confront the corruption of privilege.

There had been warnings to be sure! In 1979 I wrote an editorial for the *Journal of the Irish Colleges of Physicians and Surgeons* in which I proposed a combination of the College of Physicians in Kildare Street and the College of Surgeons on

Stephen's Green. Both colleges served the common interest of undergraduate and postgraduate medicine in Ireland, occupying two buildings within a quarter of a mile's distance from each other, with duplication of staff and facilities. I suggested selling the College of Physicians to the adjoining National Library of Ireland, and relocating the facility on the then vacant site adjoining the College of Surgeons, so as to be able to provide superlative facilities for postgraduate medicine in Ireland.

> Is there not also a place for closer cooperation between the College of Physi-
> cians and the College of Surgeons? A businessman looking at the two colleges
> with their common interest in medical education, albeit to different groups of
> the medical fraternity, would without hesitation recommend that both should
> function from a common base, sharing educational facilities, staff, and the
> very substantial expenses involved in this age in running such institutes."[12]

While this paper was in press I was enjoying myself at the Charter Day dinner of the Royal College of Surgeons and having repaired to the gentleman's convenience at the appropriate interval I was accosted there by a triumvirate of the College hierarchy consisting of Alan Grant (then president of RCPI), Bryan Alton (then treasurer) and Ciaran Barry (then registrar, who manned the door so as to prevent entry from other guests) and was advised to withdraw the article, which they found offensive to the College. I argued that rather than do so it would be more appropriate for one, or all of them, to write a response putting forward the College's case rebutting my proposal. The following day I received a phone call from a senior colleague, who had proposed me for the fellowship of the College many years earlier, advising me strongly to withdraw the article. I refused to do so and the editorial was published without either supportive or derogatory comment, which underlies the futility of censorship efforts.

But there were to be further ominous signs. To highlight the bicentenary of the Royal College of Surgeons in 1984 I wrote a paper in the *British Medical Journal*[13] (which was also published in the *Journal of the Irish Colleges of Surgeons and Physicians*)[14] praising the College for its achievements over two centuries but also criticizing the academic staff for lacking the vision of their counterparts in Britain and America, where professorial departments were devoted not only to teaching, but also to research. A number of College graduates viewed this 'with great displeasure' in a letter to the College journal,[15] which was fair enough, but when the editor declined to publish my response to the graduates, I wrote to him pointing out that he had once again allowed the establishment to stifle opinion that was contrary to its perceived position of righteousness:

By allowing yourself to become arbiter of polemical issues, you are in my view supporting what has been establishment policy in Dublin medicine for too long, namely the earnestly held belief that establishment opinion is infallible and anything distasteful or contrary to it must be negated. Surely, honesty and the freedom to express a view-point, which is after all the corner stone of democracy, should be the guiding light for editors?[16]

Two years later I was to be made acutely aware of how naively idealistic these sentiments were and how in reality freedom of speech is something of an oxymoron in Irish medicine. In 1987, as editor of the *Irish Medical Journal*, I wrote an editorial entitled 'Strike and the Medical Profession' criticizing doctors for having resorted to strike in pursuit of solving their grievances and argued for alternative ways by which issues of contention between the government and the profession could be resolved.[17] As a cardiologist in charge of a coronary care unit, I was well placed to witness first-hand the serious consequences of withdrawal of service from the acutely ill and I was also convinced of the absolute futility of the exercise. This caused such distress to the Irish Medical Organization (a trade union and proprietor of the journal) that rather than dismiss me as editor (which might have been contestable in court) the Organization took the expedient of closing the journal on the grounds that it was losing money, and re-opened it under a new editor some months later.[18]

The event attracted international scrutiny. The *British Medical Journal* pointed out that 'O'Brien made it clear that he was willing to publish letters opposing his views on strike, and the last issue of the journal contained two such letters. It also contained fifteen letters deploring the closure of the journal, many of them coming from the most prestigious names in Irish medicine ... But to return to the case in question, given that in Eoin O'Brien there is an editor as well as a cardiologist of international repute, should a country that has produced Grattan, Burke, and Connolly – not to mention Swift, Shaw, and Yeats – not think again?'[19] The editor of the *Journal of the American Medical Association* saw the 'tragic demise of the *Irish Medical Journal* ... after fifty years of publication' as 'a sad example of what can happen when there are severe conflicts between the medical organization owner and an editor exercising freedom'.[20] In fact the American journal went on to devote three pages to examining the background to the journal's closure.[21] The conservative *Lancet* gave an interesting analysis: 'The very first editorial (in 1937) spoke of the hope to 'make the journal a medium for free expression.'[22] It is ironic that the free expression of the last editor, Dr Eoin O'Brien, should have created such a furore; his final editorial, the traditional Irish speech from the dock, is sad reading. 'O'Brien's views on strikes by the medical profession are, alas, becoming unfashionable. In fact, with the increasing trade-unionization of the profession they are out of date. O'Brien's dissent has become too big a bone of contention to bury.'[23]

Strike and the Medical Profession, 1987

THE RECENT STRIKE by non-consultant hospital doctors raises many issues that need to be deliberated upon lest the profession should ever contemplate embarking on such a course again. First, any form of industrial action in the medical profession carries the potential for causing considerable hardship and harm to those very people doctors are there to serve, namely their patients, and the deleterious effects of such action must be carefully balanced against potential gains.

However justifiable a sense of grievance may have been among the non-consultant hospital doctors – and they were by no means alone in the profession in experiencing the effects of the recent financial cutbacks – the issues on which their strike action was based were far from clear. They certainly did not justify the ultimate weapon of withdrawal of service, when forceful negotiation, backed up if necessary by other forms of industrial action, might have achieved the same result.

The consequences of the strike were felt by patients (though the effects were minimized by the participation of consultants in maintaining the hospital services), general practitioners, who had to contend with the increased work load consequent upon the closure of out-patients and accident and emergency departments, consultants, nurses, para-medical workers and the administrative staffs in the hospitals, all of whom had to contribute in differing proportions to maintaining a limited hospital service for the public.

The effect of the strike on many non-consultant hospital doctors was also none too pleasant. Some of the few who chose to ignore the call to strike, because their principles dictated otherwise, were subject to considerable personal conflict and on occasion to pressure that was not far removed from the intimidatory practices associated with the more militant fringe of trade unionism. The personal anguish caused to many of those who went on strike against their better principles was also considerable. The Medical Council had to deliberate long and hard on the consequences of the strike for provisionally registered doctors and had the strike been protracted, the Medical Council might have had no alternative but to withhold registration for many doctors. Then there was the effect on the medical profession as a whole. The public image of the profession is dependent upon the behaviour of its members, and strike, which is regarded by many as anathema to doctors, demeans the profession as a whole and blurs the distinction between a profession and a trade; words the very meaning of which derive from a code of practice rather than being, as some would have it, a mere semantic quibble. Though many of the more militant non-consultant hospital doctors would place little value on such sentiments, even they would have to agree that the recent strike was a failure, and whatever meagre gains might be attributed to it did not justify the terrible risk inherent in such action.

The strike has highlighted differing attitudes in the profession, namely that on the one hand there are doctors who are prepared to strike, some for relatively paltry gain and others only if provoked beyond what they consider to be endurance, and then there are those who will never strike because they consider it morally indefensible for a doctor to withhold his service from a sick person. The former subscribe to the belief that strike action is justifiable if it sustains a secure profession, which will ultimately be beneficial to society. Doctors opposed to strike believe that regardless of the difficulties they may encounter with government departments, they can never jeopardize their patient's welfare by withholding their services. They evaluate their position, moreover, not merely in terms of finance, but see themselves as privileged in having been afforded a period of intellectual development in training for a profession that commands a position of esteem in society, in return for which, standards, often difficult to maintain, are demanded. Comparisons with, for example, the hourly rate paid to other workers are not seen by doctors holding this view as valid because all such analogies fail to measure the considerable satisfaction that is the reward, often the only one, for simply being a good doctor. Nor do such comparisons take account of the many varied opportunities that a career in medicine offers. In the face of the assertive form of collective action that characterized the recent strike, doctors morally opposed to such a course were denied an opportunity to express an opinion and they remained, for the greater part, silent. Their presence must now be recognized, not so much by way of a catharsis, nor merely to assess their numerical presence (which is unknown but may be considerable), nor indeed as a means of tempering opposing views (which being antithetical are irreconcilable though one may in the course of time influence the other), but in recognition of the fundamental ethic of the medical profession that puts the patient before all other considerations.

There are lessons, therefore, to be learned from this strike. First, in Ireland, as in other countries where strike in the medical profession has also failed, strike action should not be a stratagem in industrial negotiation. It should be clear to all but the most politically myopic that government will no longer permit privileged groups to dictate policy and that to do so is effectively a denigration of the democratic process. This being so, the profession should give careful consideration to foregoing the right to strike in return for which it would obtain a guarantee of responsible and prompt negotiation with efficient arbitration procedures. If the profession ever considers resorting to strike again it must not do so without a mandate from the *entire* profession. It is unacceptable for a group such as the non-consultant hospital doctors to inflict chaos in other sectors of the profession without obtaining the support of those groups. In future all doctors, the recently qualified and provisionally registered, the non-consultant hospital doctors, the consultants, the general practitioners, and all other groupings of doctors within the profession must be balloted on the advisability or otherwise of strike action. Had such a course been taken prior to the last strike it is probable that the unhappy event would not have occurred.

Medical Journalism

JOURNALISM OFFERED ME the *modus operandi* that permitted thoughts to be expressed, concepts to be aired and debate stimulated. Journalism taught me that putting one's thoughts into words may invite invective and that to assume, as I once did, that an expressed opinion would receive reasoned debate from a liberal and educated profession that might be expected to uphold freedom of speech was often not the case. Whatever personal hurt my forays into medical journalism may have brought I have no regrets, because by declaring my views, I was permitted to express misgivings and to highlight what I believed to be important issues in medicine.

My introduction to medical journalism began when I was appointed registrar to Alex Paton in Dudley Road Hospital (now the City Hospital) in Birmingham in October 1968. I attribute this appointment to just one feature of my then meagre curriculum vitae, namely a publication in *The Lancet* entitled 'Inhibition of Antiplasmin and Fibrinolytic Effect of Protease in Patients with Cancer',[24] which earned editorial comment.[25] Alex Paton tutored me in general medicine with a bias towards gastroenterology; he also taught me a lesson in what might be called the realism of humility. In March 1971 I took a week's holiday and came across to Dublin to successfully sit the membership of the Royal College of Physicians in Ireland (MRCPI). On my return to Dudley Road Hospital I went straight to Paton's office and after a few pleasantries told him I had passed my Irish membership. He shrugged his shoulders, said nothing and went back to his copy of *Current*

Contents to mark out the papers of interest to his research. A month later I went to London and successfully sat the membership of the Royal College of Physicians (MRCP). This time I entered his office a little less ebulliently than previously and reticently informed him that I had been successful in London. He rose up from his desk, took my hand and said, 'Now we're talking.' From then on he became a very potent influence in shaping my career and we soon became close friends.

In 1970 Alex introduced me to Stephen Lock, who was then a staff editor of the *British Medical Journal* (later to become editor for sixteen years), and this led to my being recruited as a reporter for the journal by Dougal Swinscow, who was deputy editor (and a lichenologist of repute). My first assignment was to report on the Annual Scientific Meeting of the British Medical Association at the Royal Baths Assembly Rooms in Harrogate. Here I joined a small group of reporters that included Bill Whimster, Bertie Wood and Jim Petrie. We travelled much together over a five-year period under the watchful eye of either Stephen Lock or the late Richard Smith, had much fun and became good friends. The format of reportage was rigid and allowed for no personal form of expression, and when we tried to sneak in a mischievous sentence reflecting our individuality it was invariably edited out before the hand-written copy was sent by train to London for printing. The following are examples taken at random from meetings I reported on during this period:

> Fourteenth Annual Clinical Meeting of the British Medical Association, Aberyswyth, 1–4 April 1971: 'With Mr A.S. Alms (Cardiff) in the chair the opening contribution to a symposium on the patient's part in healing was given by Canon M.A. Hugh Melinsky (Norwich), who stated that he firmly believed that the patient had a contribution to make in the healing process. Why some patients succumbed to an illness whereas others did not was a fascinating problem. In such a discussion it was difficult to draw dividing lines between the mind, body, and soul. Illness frequently protected the body against the insults of life, excellent examples being shellshock in war and the fainting Victorian maiden who found the pressures of the drawing room more than she could tolerate ... Mr J.R. Bambrough (Dean, St John's College, Cambridge) discussing medicine and secular morality opened by recounting a story in which the master of a Cambridge college, a man of strong Tory and Anglican principles, had interviewed a young student and had shown him a map of England with many shaded areas; on being asked the significance of these shaded areas the student, after much deliberation, replied that they represented areas that returned Labour members to Parliament; the master, obviously well pleased, stated that though this was not the correct answer it had been the best he had yet received – the shaded areas in fact represented

the areas of opposition to vaccination against smallpox in the nineteenth century.'[26]

Jamaica Medical Congress – Seventeenth Annual Clinical Meeting of the British Medical Association in conjunction with the Medical Association of Jamaica, Kingston, Jamaica, 21–27 April 1974: 'Dr Michael DeBakey (USA) then gave the 1974 Winthrop Lecture on recent advances in the management of coronary artery disease, a subject of great magnitude, common to all parts of the world. After studying 10,000 coronary arteriograms over fifteen years, he considered that the patterns of the disease could now be seen in two ways. Firstly, occlusive disease could affect the larger arteries leaving the distal ones unimpaired; this could be relieved by operation, such as venous bypass graft or by endarterectomy. But if the distal vascular bed was impaired, a less common occurrence, no medical or surgical methods were available to relieve it. Secondly, patients differed in the rate at which occlusive lesions progressed – though in only 25% of patients was the progression rapid. Turning to risk factors, in his series about 80% of the patients had smoked, 40% were hypertensive, 40% had abnormalities of lipoprotein metabolism, and 15% had diabetes.'[27]

Occasionally it was possible to escape the rigid format of reportage and give a more personal view of the meetings of the British Medical Association as I was able to do in the *Irish Medical Journal* for the East Mediterranean Medical Congress – Fifteenth Annual Clinical Meeting of the British Medical Association in Cyprus, 11–15 April 1972:

The East Mediterranean Medical Congress, incorporating the 15th Annual Clinical Meeting of the British Medical Association was officially opened in the Municipal Theatre, Nicosia by His Beatitude Archbishop Makarios, president of Cyprus on Wednesday, 12th April 1972. If I ever return to Cyprus, I will stay at Kyrenia, a beautiful seaside town situated on the north shore, and encircling a picturesque harbour, which is not unlike an Irish fishing village; towering above the harbour is the impressive 13th century Kyrenia castle. However, the main attraction for me, was the indescribable beauty of Bellapais Abbey (Abbey of Peace), situated in the hills within a few miles of Kyrenia at a height of one thousand feet; this 14th century monastery is one of the finest examples of Gothic architecture in the Middle East and commands a view of the surrounding countryside, which must be second to none. The Gothic cloisters, the flowers, the birds and the view blend to produce an atmosphere of tranquillity and serenity, which must be conducive to holiness. Laurence Durrell certainly chose a magnificent place to write *Bitter Lemons*.

The medical highlight of the congress was, for me, the clinical demonstration at the British Military Hospital in Dhekelia. Finally six patients with leprosy were presented; here I saw what had previously been but a textbook impression – the lepromatous, borderline and tuberculoid forms of leprosy, the hypopigmented and hyperesthetic dermal lesions, the thickened palpable peripheral nerves, muscular atrophy, severe joint deformities, and the classical 'leonine facies' and saddle nose. The tragedy of Hansen's disease, as one of the doctors at Dhekelia told me, is that for as little as five shillings the disease can be arrested with dapsone.[28]

My involvement as a reporter with the *British Medical Journal* in turn led to an invitation to write a number of unsigned editorials for the journal. Stephen Lock always liked pithy titles for these editorials and if they drew on literature as in 'Or in the Heart or in the Head'[29] and 'Will No-One Tell Me What She Sings?'[30] so much the better. However, when I submitted an editorial inspired by the death of a French bishop in a brothel with a title with which I was much pleased – 'The Bishop in the Bordello' – prurient editorship in keeping with the mores of the times saw this title modified to 'Coitus and Coronaries'[31] with all reference to the libidinous bishop being removed. At the same time Dr Harry Counihan, who was editor of the *Journal of the Irish Medical Association*, invited me to write editorials for his journal. In 1975 Stephen Lock commissioned a series of articles for the *British Medical Journal* 'on events medical and otherwise in Ireland' and a series of articles were published under 'The Letter From Dublin' title over three years or so. In 1978 Harry Counihan commissioned a series of articles under the curious title 'Kincoran Opinion', which were published in the *Journal of the Irish Medical Association*. In the essay 'Stephen Lock – Hibernain in Disguise' (written on the occasion of Stephen's retirement as editor of the *British Medical Journal*) I pay tribute to the potent influences of literature, conversation and medical journalism.[32]

When I returned to Ireland from the UK my freelance journalistic experience was channelled into the more formal roles of journal editorship. I was appointed editor of the *Journal of the Irish Colleges of Physicians and Surgeons* from 1973 until 1976, and took up the reigns as editor of this journal again from 1988 to 1993. The Irish Medical Association invited me to become editor of the *Irish Medical Journal* in 1986, a short-lived tenure for reasons that have been previously discussed. In my role as editor of these journals I sought to marry art and medicine by illustrating the covers of the journals with relevant paintings and photographs and by encouraging articles on the history of medicine and the place of the humanities and humanitarian considerations in the medical curriculum.

I enjoyed medical journalism in its different guises and I was privileged to be able to examine, and who knows perhaps influence, the progress of medicine, but I was alas brought face-to-face with one of the profession's most serious shortcomings, namely its inability to brook criticism of its performance and behaviour. Perhaps this intolerance to criticism was all the more unpalatable coming from a journalist within the profession rather than would have been the case if such comment had emanated from without.

Stephen Lock: Hibernian in Disguise, 1991

THERE ARE, as I see it, two facets to friendship. The bond of affection, fundamental to all friendship, determines the intensity and durability of the relationship; it need not trouble us here – it is of now, personal and enduring. The influence deriving from a friendship on the lives that form the union is in many ways more complex, being for the greater part beyond the control of the protagonists; the ripples and waves emanating from my friendship with Stephen Lock have buoyed the craft of my existence through many strata of life and learning.

We met in 1970 in – of all places – the Royal Baths Assembly Rooms at Harrogate on the occasion of the British Medical Association Annual Clinical Meeting when he was an assistant editor and I a novice reporter, then registrar to Alex Paton in Birmingham. Here began reportage à la BMJ: 'Speaking on the dangers of thought in medical education, Professor Rudmose Glaring emphasized that the aim of all medical school curricula should be to provide so comprehensive a programme of teaching that the luxury of thought on the part of the student would be quite unnecessary.' And on and on we would go, even in our sleep, as indeed was often the case. To Southampton, Jamaica, Cyprus – in the reign of His Beatitude the President of the Republic, Archbishop Makarios – to Aberystwyth and elsewhere, not now remembered. No harm in that, as such is not my brief. How to depict, in a manner appropriate to the occasion, Stephen Lock's long and varied association with Ireland is the task at hand. What a kaleidoscope of memories from this country where Stephen is, perhaps, most at home. I will use the music of this island – its literature – to illustrate his love of Ireland and its people. To others must fall the task of illuminating his involvement with opera.

At Renvyle after dinner, sometime in 1976 I think, the subject was Joyce, the decision arrived at was that he could only be appreciated to the full and indeed understood when read aloud; and so into the small hours:

Can't hear with the waters of. The chittering waters of. Flittering bats, field-mice bawk talk. Ho! Are you not going ahome? What Thom Malone? Can't hear with bawk of bats, all thim liffeying waters of. Ho, talk save us! My foos

THE WEIGHT OF COMPASSION & OTHER ESSAYS

woon't moos. I feel as old as yonder elm. A tale told of Shaun or Shem? All
Livia's daughtersons. Dark hawks hear us. Night! Night! My ho head halls. I
feel as heavy as yonder stone. Tell me of John or Shaun? Who were Shem and
Shaun the living sons or daughters of? Night now! Tell me, tell me, tell me,
elm! Nighty night! Telmetale of stem or stone. Beside the rivering waters of,
hitherandthithering waters of. Night!

On to Lissadell, another Irish writer, this time a poet – aren't they all? To sit
in the bay window of the Georgian house, then slowly decaying, and recall times
past with melancholy:

> The light of evening, Lissadell,
> Great windows open to the south,
> Two girls in silk kimonos, both
> Beautiful, one a gazelle.
> But a raving autumn shears
> Blossom from the summer's wreath;
> The older is condemned to death,
> Pardoned, drags out lonely years
> Conspiring among the ignorant.
> I know not what the younger dreams –Some
> vague Utopia – and she seems,
> When withered old and skeleton-gaunt,
> An image of such politics.
> Many a time I think to seek
> One or the other out and speak
> Of that old Georgian mansion, mix
> Pictures of the mind, recall
> That table and the talk of youth,
> Two girls in silk kimonos, both
> Beautiful, one a gazelle.

At Thoor Ballylee, at another time, a dissertation by Dr Lock on Yeats's reju-
venation following the Steinach operation undergone by Yeats in 1934:

> How can I, that girl standing there,
> My attention fix
> On Roman or on Russian
> Or on Spanish politics? [...]
> And maybe what they say is true
> Of war and war's alarms
> But O that I were young again
> And held her in my arms!

One sun-drenched day in Monkstown under cherry blossom, destined to bloom no more than three weeks each year, a group caught in the time-frame of memory recited Yeats and Gogarty. One, Niall Sheridan, rose with his glass in the lengthening evening shadow and querulously asked if any of the assembled company were aware that the inspiration for the closing lines of 'Ringsend' was Lapsang Souchong tea, once, but happily not now, a most popular beverage in Dublin:

> I will live in Ringsend
> With a red-headed whore,
> And the fanlight gone in
> Where it lights the hall-door,·
> And listen each night
> For her querulous shout
> As at last she streels in
> And the pubs empty out.
> To soothe that wild breast
> With my old-fangled songs,
> Till she feels it redressed
> From inordinate wrongs,
> Imagined, outrageous,
> Preposterous wrongs,
> Till peace at last comes,
> Shall be all I will do,
> Where the little lamp blooms
> Like a rose in the stew;
> And up the back garden
> The sound comes to me
> Of the lapsing, unsoilable,
> Whispering sea.

What is the stuff of poetry spake one? When is art asked another? Ah! Here was the stuff of conversation whatever of poetry. Poetry, art or neither cried another?

> We are the masturbators
> We are the dreamers of dreams
> Spending in secretive places,
> Our totally purposeless streams;
> And one with a mind at leisure
> Can roger an ancient Queen
> And make from a moment's pleasure
> A map on the damascene.

And the written word. Its beauty. Its elusiveness. How to hold it, mercurial, in the cup of one's hand and how to thread the words into the whole that is art. Compare, says one, the first published 'Leda' in *To-morrow* in 1924 with the revised version. Were they the same poem?

> A rush, a sudden wheel and hovering still
> The bird descends, and her frail thighs are pressed
> By the webbed toes, and that all powerful bill
> Has laid her helpless face upon his breast.
> How can those terrified vague fingers push
> The feathered glory from her loosening thighs!
> All the stretched body's laid on the white rush
> And feels the strange heart beating where it lies;
> A shudder in the loins engenders there
> The broken wall, the burning roof and tower
> And Agamemnon dead.
>   Being so caught up,
> So mastered by the brute blood of the air,
> Did she put on his knowledge with his power
> Before the indifferent beak could let her drop?

And then the revised version published in *The Tower* in 1928:

> A sudden blow: the great wings beating still
> Above the staggering girl, her thighs caressed
> By the dark webs, her nape caught in his bill,
> He holds her helpless breast upon his breast.
>
> How can those terrified vague fingers push
> The feathered glory from her loosening thighs?
> And how can body, laid in that white rush,
> But feel the strange heart beating where it lies?
>
> A shudder in the loins engenders there
> The broken wall, the burning roof and tower
> And Agamemnon dead.
>   Being so caught up,
> So mastered by the brute blood of the air,
> Did she put on his knowledge with his power
> Before the indifferent beak could let her drop?

And when it all became too much an early morning catharsis at the Forty Foot where nudity strips not only clothes but all pretence of class, creed and culture.

The postman, the milkman, the unemployed, literati, university dons, clerics of all denominations – all defrocked, and on one memorable morning, a cabal of medical editors from diverse corners of the globe, were as one in the scrotum-tightening waters of this freezing bathing hole, which had been chosen for the opening scene of *Ulysses*:

> Stately, plump Buck Mulligan came from the stairhead bearing a bowl of lather on which a mirror and a razor lay crossed. A yellow dressing gown, ungirdled, was sustained gently behind him on the mild morning air. He held the bowl aloft and intoned:
> – *Introibo ad altare Dei.*
> Halted, he peered down the dark winding stairs and called out coarsely:
> – Come up, Kinch! Come up, you fearful Jesuit!
> Solemnly he came forward and mounted the round gunrest. He faced about and blessed gravely thrice the tower, the surrounding country and the awakening mountains.

Stephen, at home where the boundaries of thought were being at least probed, if not nudged forward, intrigued by the Irishman's desire to dance on the edge of the volcano, despondent but not surprised when talent was consumed by the fires, was lulled to peace in such places as Coole, where the lake's shy swans drifted towards us many years ago:

> The trees are in their autumn beauty
> The woodland paths are dry,
> Under the October twilight the water
> Mirrors a still sky;
> Upon the brimming water among the stones
> Are nine and fifty swans.
> The nineteenth autumn has come upon me
> Since I first made my count,
> I saw, before I had well finished
> All silently mount
> And scatter wheeling in great broken rings
> Upon their clamorous wings.

Our times together at Thoor Ballylee, Coole, Ben Bulben, Drumcliffe, Renvyle, de Vesci and Clifton Terrace hopefully weave as pleasant memories for Stephen as for me. May our paths join here some summer morning at the Forty Foot where we once swam, as did others before us, as will others long after we have been. Until then I know I speak for his many friends in Ireland in saluting Stephen Lock's mighty international contribution to medical journalism and in acknowledging with sincerity his friendship for this country and in particular our friendship, which includes also Shirley and Tona. Our wishes are for the success and happiness that marked his association with the BMJ to be also the attributes of his newly chosen career.

Humanitarian Involvement

ANOTHER POTENT INFLUENCE – humanitarianism – has moulded my attitude to the broader dimensions of medicine. A remarkable friend, Kevin Cahill, whom I first met in or around 1973, introduced me to the world of humanitarian affairs. Kevin was a close friend of Harry O'Flanagan, who was then registrar of the Royal College of Surgeons in Ireland. Due to Harry's prescience in recognizing that a medical school with international alumni must at least acknowledge the plight of poorer countries, Kevin was appointed professor of tropical medicine (a post he was to occupy for thirty-five years). I had just been appointed acting professor of pharmacology and therapeutics and we both met frequently to discuss our mutual interests in medicine and literature. Kevin had travelled extensively in the humanitarian cause, having served as director of clinical tropical medicine in Egypt and Sudan while in the US navy and he had continued active medical research in Africa, Latin America, and the Near and Far East, with service in Somalia, Sudan, India, and Nicaragua. Kevin introduced me to a world of medicine that had never been even mentioned, much less studied, during my six-year apprenticeship in an institution that boasted of its international influence.

In 1992 Kevin founded The Center for International Humanitarian Co-operation (CIHC, which now has non-governmental organization [NGO] status) to promote healing and peace in countries shattered by natural disasters, armed conflicts, and ethnic violence. He asked me to join the Board where I met a group of people willing to give of their time, energy and resources to foster and encourage humanitarian assistance in strife-torn areas of the world. These remarkable people, who became close friends, included the late Paul Hamlyn, publisher and benefactor who established the Paul Hamlyn Foundation in 1987 – one of the UK's largest independent grant-giving organizations – as a focus for his charitable interests, but whose personal attributes of kindness, humour and generosity cannot be conveyed in the brevity of a sentence. Paul's widow Helen, a woman of remarkable enterprise and energy, has succeeded her husband on the Board; the late Cyrus Vance who had been United States secretary of state during Jimmy Carter's presidency; Boutros Boutros-Ghali, secretary-general of the United Nations in 1992; Peter Tarnoff, president of the International Advisory Corporation based in San Francisco and a former career Foreign Service Officer in the US Department of State; Daniel Boyer, a Serb whose villa in Geneva served as a discussion point for the Vance-Owen peace accord for the former Yugoslavia in 1993; Rev. Joseph A. O'Hare, S.J. who was President Emeritus of Fordham University from 1984 to 2003, the longest tenure as president in the 164-year history of the University; Abdulrahim Abby Farah, who served for twenty years as under-secretary-general and senior political advisor on African affairs in the United Nations; David Owen, physician and neurologist, a member of parliament for twenty-six years during which time he was navy minister, health minister, and foreign secretary. Jan Eliasson, lately the United Nations secretary-general special representative for mediation in the Darfur crisis, and formerly Sweden's ambassador to the US and to the UN; Peter Hansen, who retired from the United Nations after twenty-eight years of service, the last nine as commissioner-general of the UN Relief and Works Agency which provided education, health, relief and social services to more than 3.2 million registered Palestinian refugees living in Jordan, Lebanon, Syria, the West Bank, and the Gaza Strip; Francis Mading Deng, UN special adviser to the secretary-general on the prevention of genocide, and Richard Goldstone, the former chief prosecutor of the UN International War Crimes Tribunal for the former Yugoslavia and Rwanda. The essay 'The Tragedy of the Medicine Man in the Underdeveloped World' written as long ago as 1989, is a gesture of acknowledgment to the humanitarian achievements of Kevin Cahill. [33]

When I joined the CIHC one of the Center's main aims was to add momentum to the increasing demand for an international ban on landmines. Landmines have been described by the US Department of State as the most toxic and widespread pollution facing mankind. Landmines are vicious weapons and their makers have no hesitation in incorporating the latest technology to improve them so as to inflict even greater mutilation and suffering on their victims. There are blast mines, fragmentation mines, butterfly mines, bounding mines, mines with anti-handling devices to kill those who try to defuse them, and smart mines that can be reprogrammed to self-detonate (but as many as half fail to do so, leaving the need for conventional mine clearance). Mines can be laid by hand or by remote delivery; they can be scattered over wide areas from artillery or rocket warheads, aircraft or helicopters, which can disperse as many as 2000 mines in a few minutes.

I was privileged to be able to visit the Sawai Man Singh Hospital in Jaipur, where the 'Jaipur foot', a simple but ingenious and inexpensive prosthesis was developed for Indian amputees, whose injuries usually result from falling from trains. But now the Jaipur foot is in demand in many mined countries, where its low price and simplicity of production (often by trained local amputees) and its durability make it suited to the circumstances of developing countries where the people often go barefooted and work in damp rugged conditions. The essay 'Walk in peace: Banish Landmines from our Globe' [34] is one of the many essays I wrote on this topic.

Quite apart from the landmines tragedy, Kevin led me along many unfamiliar paths, not least being one that led me to the United Nations to speak on the diplomatic implications of emerging diseases in a symposium on preventive diplomacy.[35] He also persuaded me to write the essay 'Human Rights and the Making of a Good Doctor' for a book he edited, *Traditions, Values and Humanitarian Action*, in which I attempt to put the case for humanitarianism being a mandatory part of the curricula of all medical schools. [36]

In recent years the CIHC has concentrated on the educational needs of humanitarian workers in crisis-afflicted areas of the world. Towards this end the Center established the International Diploma in Humanitarian Assistance (IDHA). This practical comprehensive course enables aid workers and their organizations to function more effectively and efficiently in times of war or following natural calamities. The IDHA community now numbers over 990 graduates from over 120 nations, the great majority of whom are aid workers with field experience. IDHA graduates and faculty represent most UN agencies, as well as all major non-governmental humanitarian organizations, and military, diplomatic, academic, political, and religious groups from around the world. [37]

Attention to humanitarian issues in medicine not only opens up a vision of a world in turmoil, but also suggests that giving a little of what one has gained from medicine can influence change for the better for those who are deprived of the most basic necessities. When in 1992 Dr Shanthi Mendis, then co-ordinator of The Chronic Diseases Prevention and Management Department of Chronic Diseases at WHO invited me to co-chair with her a committee of experts to specify the criteria for a device to measure blood pressure in the poorer countries of the world, I accepted immediately. Working with a group of friends and colleagues we have engaged the manufacturing industry to produce a simple, inexpensive, robust and accurate solar powered device with which we hope to alleviate the burden of disease being caused by high blood pressure in low resource countries, especially by reducing the awful toll of maternal mortality in pregnancy. [38]

The Tragedy of the Medicine Man in the Underdeveloped World, 1989

IT IS, PERHAPS, not entirely a coincidence that Kevin Cahill's book *A Bridge to Peace* should arrive for review at the same time as the *Journal* publishes the proceedings of the first overseas meeting of the Royal College of Surgeons in Ireland in Bahrain, as well as a paper by a young surgeon on his experiences in Ghana and a review of female circumcision in underdeveloped countries. Nor is it entirely without coincidence that the international medical literature should begin at last to consider seriously the condition of humanity in the underdeveloped world. One of the most regrettable features of postgraduate medical education, be it medical or surgical, in western society has been the virtual penalization of the idealistic young doctor who sets out either to broaden his or her experience, or sometimes seeks merely to repay to society something in return for the privilege he or she perceives a career in medicine to be. How galling it has been for such doctors to see the laurels of success awarded to colleagues who chose to play it safe by staying close to home and following the conservative course to success as enunciated by the Royal Colleges.

This is the tragedy of the Medicine Man in the underdeveloped world, but though the tragedy may be his or hers (in the short term at any rate), the dishonour for such a policy must rest fairly and squarely with the postgraduate educational authorities. Happily, there is now evidence that doctors who chose to spend some time working in underdeveloped areas, for whatever reason, may indeed turn the experience to advantage in furthering their career prospects.

Of greater interest, however, is the possibility that experience gained by these doctors in poor and neglected countries, where exploitation by the nations whence they come is the order of the day, will give them the ability not only to see at first hand the corruption that is around them, and to sense, perhaps for the first time, the essence of evil, but also the courage to speak frankly and fearlessly of their experiences. In so doing they may achieve more because of their privileged position than journalists and other observers can ever hope to do. This role may be further enhanced by the doctor's proximity to power and with this there comes, on occasion, the opportunity to influence for the better the course of history. If this unique position, which may only be attained by a relatively small, but none-theless significant, proportion of the profession, is to be used for the betterment of mankind. It may seem superfluous to add that any such outcome is wholly dependent on integrity. And yet it is not superfluous to do so because, paradoxi-cally, the attainment of a position of influence necessitates exposure to corruption.

None is more aware of these conflicting forces than Kevin Cahill. He has felt the heat of the political fire in his role as director of health services in New York City. In his capacity as professor of tropical medicine at the Royal College of Surgeons, director of the Tropical Disease Center at Lennox Hill Hospital, consultant to the United Nations Medical Service, and a member of the Council on Foreign Relations, he has worked in Somalia, Libya and Nicaragua. He has not only written about his experiences, he has had the courage to criticize American policy in Nicaragua at a time when such criticism was deemed almost unpatriotic at home. Dr Cahill is dismissive of this, claiming that it took 'little courage' to identify with those who suffer and die for freedom. Not all would see it thus.

A Bridge to Peace is a collection of Dr Cahill's essays written over the period 1982–1987 for papers and periodicals such as the *New York Times* and the *Journal of the Irish Colleges of Physicians and Surgeons*. A major theme to the book is that the doctor has a unique opportunity to observe mankind in conflict and deprivation and to utilize his skill and experience to formulate reasoned judgment which, with the erudition that should be part and parcel of his persona, he may use to influence public opinion.

If the foundations of Dr Cahill's thesis are medicine, an appreciation of the humanities, integrity and courage, the *Bridge* itself is compassion. This sentiment is applied ruthlessly, but not, in my view, excessively, to destroy the cant of political expediency that ignores the horror of personal suffering; it is brought to bear not only on the conflicts in the unfortunate countries of which Dr Cahill has first-hand working experience but also to explore some not well-recognized aspects of Irish-American relations on Northern Ireland (Dr Cahill is president of the American Irish Historical Society), and to plead to society for more tolerance and understanding for the disadvantaged victims of the AIDS epidemic.

To put Dr Cahill's credentials in perspective for the rather onerous task he has taken upon himself it is best to proceed directly to Maestro Leonard Bernstein's tribute to his friend, which characteristically is hidden at the back of the book rather than forming, as custom would decree, a preface or foreword. Bernstein sees him as a complicated creature 'once called a "Medicine Man", a term that presents us with a host of dualities: pillar of society/leprechaun; medieval alchemist/ medical master; shaman/clinician; witchdoctor/psychologist; juggler/saint'. In his friend, the physician Bernstein identifies something that may be fundamental to the 'Medicine Man', an appreciation of the diversity of activity that makes existence so complex but at the same time renders it tolerable. An appreciation of art is but one example of which Bernstein writes: 'And Kevin sometimes comes to my concerts, and acts as if he really enjoys them, although my guess is that he knows as much about Mahler as I do about salmonella.'

Whether he understands Mahler or not is irrelevant to Bernstein, what is important is that the mind in pursuit of experience beyond the mundane is at worst a tolerant one and at best may be inspirational. Either way the ability of such an individual to listen, comprehend and then advise is the essence of the 'Medicine Man'. For Bernstein *A Bridge to Peace* is 'a kind of prayer book or breviary – a Mass applicable to any faith, or even non-faith'. A moving tribute indeed from the high altar of art, and yet only one example that serves to emphasize Dr Cahill's point that the good physician should be a much-loved man – Bernstein cannot banish the word 'love' from his essay. Indeed Kevin Cahill occupies a privileged position among writers and artists; if another example was needed one has only to turn to the dust jacket to Louis Le Brocquy's sensitive Dove of Peace painted for his friend.

There is so much to be learned from *A Bridge to Peace*, about the world in conflict, about medicine, about life and ultimately about one's self (the reader is forced to consider where he or she stands in the midst of chaos where the quality of mercy is indeed strained – surely the acid test of any book), that it should be compulsory reading for final-year medical students. For they will find in these pages descriptions of suffering and deprivation, which they can never have even imagined in the comfort of the modern teaching hospital. In Puerto Cabazas the criterion for designating a hospital area as an Intensive Care Unit is the possession of two blood pressure cuffs and a fan. Let the student consider the pathetic plight of the surgeon who refused to do any more operations without anaesthesia: 'They move too much, I just can't do it.' Here is a passage taken not quite at random:

> Statistics are a game that politicians play in war. People far from the scene are having a great debate in the American press about the accuracy of death figures in Lebanon. But there is nothing subtle about the carnage in Beirut if one can recognise or feel the feverish head of a dying child. There is no mystery about the scope of this tragedy if one walks the wards of the university hospital of the School of Theology and sees the limbless bodies, the fractured faces, the blind, the burned. These are real people, men and women and

children, hundreds of them, and no amount of sophistry can dehumanise the horrors of this war into a sterile column of figures.

The philosophy of this book is put at its pithy best by the Jesuit priest, Fr. Cesar Jerez, in his citation on the occasion of the conferring of an *honoris causa* doctorate on Dr Cahill by the Universidad Centroamericana (the only other person to be so honoured was President Carter) as 'profound Christian humanism'.

The personal message is there for each reader to do with it as he will. There is also a profound message for political leaders but unfortunately most of them don't read, or if they do, they fail to comprehend. For those in charge of medical education *A Bridge to Peace* should serve to promote a serious reappraisal of the deficiencies in the medical curriculum in relation to the underdeveloped countries of the world. But, perhaps more importantly, medical schools should give careful consideration to Dr Cahill's belief that we have at our disposal a potent resource, which we fail to use, a subject he has addressed previously in *The Untapped Resource*. It is appropriate that he should have the last word:

Public health professionals are among the most educated and, occasionally, the most respected members of a community. Yet, except when an issue impinges on their particular interest, their impact on government policy is miniscule. A physician may have the most privileged role, especially in societies where there are multiple reasons for suspicion or cynicism or even hatred. By mutual sharing, the good physician becomes part of the body and soul of the person he serves. If that trust and confidence are not abused, and if, with warmth and humility and competency, the doctor proves his worth over time, the bond becomes as durable as love. When people and nations can agree on little else, those common bonds may become the bridge to understanding and peace. There is certainly no reason not to utilize this bridge, especially in light of the dismal record of standard diplomacy.

Walk in Peace: Banish Landmines from our Globe, 1997

In Memoriam: Diana, Princess of Wales

THESE WORDS are dedicated to the memory of Diana, Princess of Wales. She, perhaps more than any other individual, in reaching out to the ravaged victims of landmines, advanced the growing demand for a total ban on these vile weapons. Her courage in exposing the hypocrisy of governments, her own included, and her compassion for the suffering in mine-infested countries, must not be to no avail. Rather it is for us to continue and to accelerate the

THE WEIGHT OF COMPASSION & OTHER ESSAYS

impetus she gave to banishing landmines from our globe, so that we can then begin to cleanse the sixty nations in which more than 100 million mines have been scattered, and permit the people – children in particular, so much loved by Diana – to walk again in peace.

The sun, deepest red at first then shimmering to gold rising over the hills of the plains, casts the father, his young son, and their dog into black relief against the sky brightening gently, imperceptibly, and reluctantly, from the dark of night to the gold of dawn. Their silhouettes slowly emerge from the darkness; the tall gaunt figure of the father, staff in one hand, a sackbag over his shoulder, the boy hopping lightly beside him holding his other hand, and the dog gambolling along between them. The father and his son are clothed scantily, both are barefoot, and their skeletal transparency betrays the hardship of chronic malnutrition. Yet the figures carry a dignity, an almost biblical majesty, as they move gracefully on their way. They are heading for a small plot from which they eke a frugal existence, that is when the crop does not fail, or war and strife do not force them to move onwards. But an uneasy stability in their region has allowed them to make this journey to their plot daily for some years.

A movement ahead attracts the dog, which darts suddenly from the man and boy to chase a field rat. The morning sky is rent with red as the body of the dog is sundered against the blueness, and the morning stillness of the plain is shattered by the blast. Before the father can react to the danger he knows so well, his son is running from the path to save his beloved dog and another ghastly blast rents the air. The father in anguish rushes headlong towards his boy, who lies moaning where he has been thrown, like a rag doll against the stump of a tree, one leg shattered. The third blast fells the father just as he reaches his son and shrapnel pierces the eyes of the boy.

As the smoke and dust settle, the scene of carnage becomes clear to the gathering villagers clustered on the edge of the path from which the trio had departed. The dog's entrails and limbs are strewn over a wide area. The boy has crawled whimpering from the tree stump, leaving a trail of blood as he drags his shattered limb along the soil. But he has reached his unconscious father, both of whose legs have disappeared. Here they lie, pathetic crumpled vestiges of humanity.

One of the younger men from the village discusses with another the path the stricken pair had taken and then advancing inch by inch; probing the ground ahead and on either side with metal rods, they slowly reach them, and as slowly drag them back, probing the ground inch by inch in reverse until they reach the path. Both father and son are now unconscious. The father is losing blood rapidly from one of his shattered legs, from which the bone protrudes obscenely. The son's leg oozes blood. The women wrap the stumps in rags moistened in a nearby rivulet from which cattle drink and in which the villagers wash. One of the men uses another piece of rag as a tourniquet to staunch the systolic ejaculations from the father's left stump.

A team of young men begin the journey to the only hospital twenty miles away. The boy is strapped to the back of one of the men and two others take the ends of a makeshift hammock on which the father is laid. This is better than a stretcher, even had such been available, as it allows them to ascend and descend the many hills between the village and their destination. Another two carry frugal supplies and some water. Ten hours later they reach the huts comprising the hospital that serves a region of some 400 square miles. The boy is in profound shock and the father is delirious.

The only surgeon in the hospital decides the boy is the more critical of the two. Two nurses tend to the father. The left leg, which had been shattered in its lower third, is now gangrenous from the tourniquet, which had not been released, and this will have to be amputated from the thigh. It may be possible to perform a below knee amputation of the right leg. The genitalia have been badly wounded by ascending shrapnel and there are a series of infected puncture wounds along the right side of the thorax. Debridement will take many hours. A unit of blood is all that the hospital can spare for the man.

The surgeon takes the young boy to theatre and looks with sadness and anger at what he has seen so often. He thinks of his own son and begins to work. The boy is shocked and dehydrated and it can be taken for granted that the wounds are severely infected. There are no intravenous antibiotics, but out of date penicillin solutions kindly donated by a charity in a far away country of affluence is administered by naso-gastric tube. The surgeon orders that two units of blood be given, even though the hospital ruling is that only one can be given in all save the most extreme emergencies: this he deems to be such. Anaesthesia like everything else being scarce, is given sparingly, and fortuitously is little needed at this stage. Apart from the shattered leg there are multiple wounds all over the frail frame. Both eyes are beyond salvage, but the shrapnel and soil must be removed. A penetrating wound like a stab wound from a knife on the left side of the jaw, on closer inspection, extends ominously into the palate and possibly further, leaving the surgeon to wonder whether, if he repairs this tragic wreck, all will be lost later from meningitis.

But he has to start and he does so with the facial and body wounds, probing for the plastic and metal components of these cruel weapons, made all the more deadly by the soil, grass and grit that contaminate them. Finally, he gives his attention to the stump, deciding that such will be the advantages to this child in future life of having a prosthesis below the knee that the risks of saving the joint are worthwhile, though he does not like the look of the badly shattered tibia that extrudes beneath the coagulated contaminated tissue. As he works he thinks of the blind child's future as a cripple. He knows only too well that as the boy grows older, the bone of the amputation stump will grow more rapidly than the surrounding skin and soft tissues and he will need multiple re-amputations. He knows that frequent infection of the amputation stump with recurrent pain will render prosthesis intolerable and add to the child's decrepitude. He asks the nurse to give more anaesthesia as he saws off the shattered bone to leave a clean sunken shaft around which he can mould the soft tissues and skin.

He has been operating for three hours. As he works he reflects that if this boy – what age could he be? No more than ten? – was to be granted a life expectancy of another forty years, which might be about right for these parts, he will probably need twenty-five prostheses in his lifetime. But the child was not so destined and he died on the operating table an hour later.

His father survived. Let us use that word literally. He survived and returned to his wife and family without his son and without his dog with scant hope of receiving even a rudimentary prosthesis, the stumps protruding hideously, a constant memory of an awful moment, a legacy from a war that had ended twelve years earlier and one in which he had not been involved other than as one of thousands who, with his family, had had to flee from one district to the next, in the ethnic wave that had swept his land. He was destined now to an even more uncertain existence than before and without a son to support him in his old age. He never laughed again, or cried, as he suffered the pains of his wounds, but it was the inner pain that scorched his mind, where it burned so incessantly as to all but consume him in its intensity. Humanity in ruins but, alas, not annihilated.

Human Rights and the Making of a Good Doctor, 2003

THE CENTRE for International Health and Co-operation was founded to promote the ethos that the physician in society can be a bridge between politicians and peace, or as an earlier publication put it, if every politician has a doctor, is this not a great 'untapped resource', a resource with the potential to influence for the good? That is assuming, of course, that the doctor in society is prepared for such a role. In *The Untapped Resource* (edited and introduced by Kevin Cahill), Hugh Carey, then a member of the US Congress, said: 'In fact, a review of our own history will show that when we had less we did more proportionately. When we were not so strong we were more generous to the weak. When we were less well fed, we helped others fend off famine.' He went on prophetically (this was 1971):

> If our country is not to act as a policeman of the world and wield the bomb as a club, then perhaps it is in our own interest and in the interest of humanity we might consider ourselves as corpsman to mankind, bearing the balm of healing and helping. Exporting our know-how in health care at relatively little cost to ourselves should be an attractive alternative to some high-cost, low-yield programs of foreign aid that we now support under the name of mutual security.

This book has within its shell three strata of discussion: 'foundations, fault lines, and corrections'. The doctor must be seen as indispensable to the 'foundations' of any tradition in humanitarian rights, and I propose to emphasize this in my essay, but more importantly, I hope to show that 'corrections' are needed, and needed urgently, if the doctor is to fulfil his potential in contributing to humanitarian action. In short, the good doctor in today's world must be versed in human rights and if this is to happen, the undergraduate student has to be taught the subject.

The doctor in society has been a figure of immense influence since the beginning of time. The physician has been portrayed in literature, music, film, and caricature, not always with kindness, but the status of the physician in society has greatly exceeded that of the other professions, probably even surpassing that of the cleric. Many assumptions are made in the portrayal of the doctor, and many commentators fail to acknowledge that a doctor is as susceptible to the failings of humankind as anyone else. Or as Shaw would have put it, 'Doctors, if no better than other men, are certainly no worse.'

The good doctor has to be all things to all men. He has to fulfil the requirements of a taxing undergraduate curriculum; he then has to undergo a postgraduate period of betterment, which, depending on his chosen specialty, can be very arduous; he must then be trusted by his patients; accepted by his peers; fulfil the dictates of the jurisdiction in which he practices; acquiesce with the dictates of his professional bodies so as to gain admission to them; and perhaps, depending on the role he casts for himself, also be a scientist and researcher prepared to write and present on his chosen avocation; be a teacher; head a large department; be an administrator; be capable of communicating with his patients, his colleagues and scientific peers; be prepared not only to keep himself abreast of advances in an ever-changing discipline but to have his knowledge and skills assessed regularly; be able to co-operate with colleagues in the delivery of health care and with colleagues abroad in the furtherance of science; be willing to work antisocial hours and to adjust his private life accordingly; he must not contract an illness that might endanger his patients' health; he must be prepared to face the medico-legal consequences for incompetence, real or imaginary; and above all, and most diffi-cultly, he must acknowledge the Socratic dictum 'Know thyself'.

Not many, one would think, could be attracted by such a job description, yet, thankfully, for society many are. My advice will add to the burden of the good doctor by calling for a further quality that carries an inevitable demand. In a world faced with humanitarian strife and with large populations in turmoil seeking refuge in stable and more prosperous nations, today's good doctor must be alert to the complex discipline of human rights, which brings the inevitable moral imperative of being aware of the prejudices that doctors, as others in society, inherit through the cultural, religious and ethnic influences of their formative environment.

I suspect more has been written on the making of a good doctor than what makes, for example, a good solicitor, fireman or accountant. Apart from numerous books, there are university courses devoted to the topic; for example, the North-eastern Ohio Universities College of Medicine offers a course over two months entitled 'In search of the Good Doctor'. The *British Medical Journal* saw the subject as one of such importance as to merit an issue devoted to 'What is a good doctor and how do you make one?' The editor accepted at the outset that his journal faced an impossible task but one that nonetheless was worth undertaking. This in-depth analysis running to some 50,000 words discusses among other relevant issues the making of a good doctor as seen from the perspective of the patient, nurses, medical students, women and doctors; it assesses the expectations of society, governing bodies and the health services, and considers the necessity for the good doctor to be able to communicate, to remain knowledgeable and skilled and to be subject to assessment of competency.

However, only in the correspondence columns (a letter from Khartoum Hospital) can any reference be found to the need for a good doctor to be aware of human rights issues: The journalist Polly Toynbee, reviewing the qualities that the General Medical Council sees as necessary in the making of a good doctor, had this to say:

> What makes the perfect modern doctor? The General Medical Council has drawn up new guidance for medical schools as a framework on which to base their curriculums and assessments. Tomorrow's Doctors is an idealistic compendium of the best qualities every new doctor should acquire. If medical schools could indeed turn out doctors moulded to this template, then we should expect a new generation of scholar saints and gentle scientists – wise, knowledgeable, sensitive, collegiate, humble, and good beyond imagining.

If human rights and humanitarian affairs seem to keep on being neglected in the making of a good doctor, such seems not to be the case with the teaching of the humanities, which has seen a remarkable resurgence in the last few decades, especially in the US. The Internet provides a truly remarkable compilation of curricula, such as the New York University online syllabi of courses in medical humanities, or the UK equivalent 'Medical Humanities Resource Database' compiled by the Centre for Health Informatics in Multiprofessional Education at University College London. The importance of this is not so much the relevance of the humanities to human rights, but rather that an awareness of the former serves as a means of bringing students close to the moral dilemmas of medicine. An acquaintance with the humanities, especially literature, imparts an appreciation of the profundity of human existence and a deeper realization of the human condition. Literature is not only enjoyable but when it enables us to discover how great writers view illness, suffering, and death it becomes an enriching formative experience.

The humanities can at least prepare the intellectual soul of the doctor-in-the-making for the tougher stuff of human rights. The artist can hone the sensitivities, kindle a desire to participate, even contribute towards the betterment of the panorama of living and dying in which the doctor is always centre-stage. The arts cannot teach us to be good human beings but they can kindle in us a desire to try to be more humane, to banish prejudice, to be kinder and more considerate. At least being aware of the contradictory influences that will confront the doctor in society places the medical student at an advantage in choosing the correct moral stance.

The need for the teaching of human rights in medical schools has been long recognized. For example, in 1992 the British Medical Association declared, 'We recommend that all medical schools incorporate medical ethics into the core curriculum and that all medical graduates make a commitment, by means of an affirmation to observe an ethical code such as the World Medical Association's (WMA) International Code of Medical Ethics.' In 1993 the General Medical Council in the UK stated that a core-objective of the undergraduate degree in medicine included a 'knowledge and understanding of ... ethical and legal issues relevant to the practice of medicine' as well as an 'awareness of the moral and ethical responsibilities involved in individual patient care'. In 1999, the WMA resolved that in so far as medical ethics and human rights form an integral part of the work and culture of the medical profession, and of the history, structure and objectives of the WMA, 'It is hereby resolved that the World Medical Association strongly recommends to Medical Schools world-wide that the teaching of Medical Ethics and Human Rights be included as an obligatory course in their curricula.'

Moreover, the United Nations has published among other documents relating to the topic 'Guidelines for national plans of action for human rights education' in which it envisages human rights education as being part of the education of 'pre-school and primary, secondary, university and other institutions of higher learning levels of education'. The many international declarations and standards on medical ethics and human rights have fallen largely on deaf ears. Despite these prestigious and authoritative mandates for the teaching of human rights to medical under-graduates, there appears to be no systematic human rights education within the curricula of the UK's twenty-seven medical schools.

Why should doctors, particularly those living in affluent stable societies, have to concern themselves with humanitarian issues? The *New Dictionary of Medical Ethics* has postulated four reasons:

> First as citizens of the modern world, they should know about the most dynamic, complex and challenging modern movement; after all, their own rights and dignity as well as those of their patients are at issue. Second, health policies, programmes and practices and clinical research may inadvertently violate human rights. Thirdly, violations of each of the rights have important adverse health effects on individuals and groups. Finally, promoting human rights is now understood as an essential part of the efforts to promote and protect public health.

No one can disagree with these recommendations, but do they go far enough? To me, there would seem to be at least three other reasons why aspiring doctors should be taught human rights. The first is that young doctors (and some old ones) are fundamentally good and even better than good, they are idealists who are often anxious to give back some of what society (or parental affluence) has given to them. Or as Shaw (who said so much so well nearly a century ago) put it:

> Unless a man is led to medicine or surgery through a very exceptional tech-nical aptitude, or because doctoring is a family tradition, or because he regards it unintelligently as a lucrative and gentlemanly profession, his motives in choosing the career of a healer are clearly generous. However actual practice may disillusion and corrupt him, his selection in the first instance is not a selection of a base character.

If the idealism of the young doctor is not exposed at least in theory to the calamities of humanitarian crises in the world and the means of alleviating them, the fire of youthful idealism is denied. A second more practical reason is that the move-ment of populations is such today that the doctor practicing even in the most settled and affluent of societies is likely to be called upon to care for displaced people.

Finally, and most importantly, the teaching of human rights should serve as a means of dispelling, or at least of bringing into focus, the prejudices that are present in us all, and which can lead to discrimination at many levels of health-care. A report to the UN Committee on Economic, Social and Cultural Rights presented alarming evidence that decisions about access to investigations and treatment in the UK are sometimes motivated by who the patients are rather than by their healthcare needs. The report highlights serious shortcomings in protecting the international right to the highest attainable standard of health, as a consequence of which some doctors discriminate against vulnerable groups, such as the elderly, prisoners, patients with HIV/AIDS, people with learning disabilities, and surprisingly, women with coronary heart disease are denied the treatment facilities afforded to men.

At an international level, the former High Commissioner for Human Rights, Mary Robinson, has identified discrimination and stigmatization as an important impediment in the global battle against HIV and AIDS.

> HIV/AIDS is one of the greatest human rights and health challenges facing the world today. HIV/AIDS-related stigma and discrimination – including discrimination in health care settings – continue to be the primary driving forces behind the epidemic by undermining prevention, treatment, care and support ... Health care professionals have a crucial role to play in ensuring respect for human rights, and the right to health and to non-discrimination in particular.

Indeed the issue of discrimination in medicine is one of considerable concern globally, and is evident not only in the UK but also in the US, in India, and no doubt in any country that cares to examine the issue.

What many doctors will not know, simply because they have never been told, is that discrimination contravenes a number of ethical codes. First, it violates the Hippocratic Oath, which anticipated human rights by nearly 2.5 millennia, and which is just as relevant to contemporary international law today as it was in 400 BC. Second, it violates one of the six non-derogable obligations within Article 12 of the International Covenant on Economic, Social and Cultural Rights, which asserts the human right of each individual to the highest attainable standard of health.

Human rights is a complex discipline in its own stead, but not one that has yet developed into a specialty in the traditional manner in medicine whereby an expert becomes a head of a department attracting others with a kindred interest to devise a suitable curriculum for undergraduate teaching. So, at least for the immediate future, even if the deans of medical schools were prepared to introduce the subject into the undergraduate curricula, most universities would simply not have the staff with the necessary interest or expertise in the subject to prepare and teach its many complexities. The British Medical Association (BMA) has examined the issue in detail by concentrating on (i) the composition and scope of ethics and human rights training; (ii) what doctors need to know; (iii) how they can obtain that knowledge, and (iv) how they can use that knowledge effectively.

As all medical schools have a course on medical ethics, the BMA begins logically by examining the mutually complementary roles of ethics and human rights. Ethics help students to understand *why* abuse should be resisted, and human rights should help them discover *what* should be done and *how* to resist abuse. Though there is considerable overlap between ethics and human rights, 'ethics teaching needs to be supplemented by human rights guidance'. Medical ethics has been taught for many years in medical schools in most countries of the world, but the quality of the course available varies greatly. Herein lies a further caveat for the teaching of human rights: the content and standard of the courses are related to the availability of teachers with the knowledge and enthusiasm to inspire their students, and various bodies have responded by producing case-based teaching packs, evaluated through workshops.

The range of material available for human rights education extends from what medical organizations produce for doctors practicing in societies in which particular human rights abuses occur. For example, the International Rehabilitation Council for Torture Victims (IRCT) based in Denmark has established training programmes dealing with the rehabilitation and care of torture survivors in Asia, the Balkans, Africa and Latin America. Likewise the Asia-Pacific Forum runs teaching programmes and rehabilitation services in Australia, Bangladesh, India, Indonesia, Nepal, New Zealand, Pakistan, Papua, New Guinea, the Philippines and Sri Lanka. Specific programmes in ethics and human rights for prison officers have been established in the former Soviet Union and Southeast Asia by the International Committee of the Red Cross. The organization International Physicians for the Prevention of Nuclear War (IPPNW) works closely with the International Federation of Medical Students, concentrating on human rights issues from the perspective of conflict prevention. Another medical student initiative, the Human Rights Union for Medical Action (HURUMA), grew out of the work undertaken in Africa by the International Federation of Medical Students and African student groups. The Commonwealth Medical Association (CMA) has developed an ethics training manual for developing countries, which integrates ethical principles and extracts from human rights conventions, with the aim of making it necessary for all health professionals to attend one training module annually as part of the requirements for renewal of the license to practice.

Moreover, the CMA has taken the innovative step of linking each statement of ethics to the provisions of the various UN human rights conventions and declarations, thereby allowing that while doctors in developing countries would not necessarily share the same cultural standards or views about medical ethics, they should nevertheless be aware of an obligation to respect the health-related human rights specified in international instruments that their governments have legally ratified.

After the fall of the Marcos regime in the Philippines in 1986, the new government made a strong commitment to promote human rights through education, and this resulted in a framework for human rights education that 'has been seen by some commentators as a useful model of who should be involved and what can be achieved'. The Consortium for Health and Human Rights with a mandate to carry out education, research and advocacy work, consists of the François-Xavier Bagnoud Center for Health and Human Rights, Global Lawyers and Physicians, Physicians for Human Rights and International Physicians for the Prevention of Nuclear War. Each of the constituent bodies of the Consortium has produced training courses in various aspects of health care and human rights. In the Netherlands, the Johannes Wier Foundation has produced a teaching module designed for doctors, nurses and paramedics, which using a case study approach places students in 'real life' situations with victims of violent crime, rape, torture and murder.

Most of the material I have referred to is designed for specific groups, or for doctors working in areas where human rights abuse is likely to occur. What is happening in the medical schools? A survey of medical schools in the UK and US showed a willingness to consider human rights in the curriculum, but there was considerable confusion between what constituted medical ethics and human rights, and overall these surveys revealed that in reality little was being taught on human rights. Indeed there is some evidence that in countries in which human rights abuses occur, the medical schools and medical organizations are active in teaching awareness of human rights, examples being Turkey, India, the Philippines, Indonesia, Malaysia and Nepal. Increasingly, the pressure and impetus for the teaching of human rights has come from medical students' organizations even though they, like their deans, are very conscious of the demands being made for more subjects to be compressed into an already overloaded curriculum. In many medical schools the students organize work experience in areas of need and deprivation, which may impart more about human rights than didactic teaching.

In the UK, Physicians for Human Rights, in conjunction with Rachel Maxwell and Derrick Pounder, has developed a cross-disciplinary course entitled 'Medicine and Human Rights', which is available free on the Internet and has been adopted by the University of Dundee as part of the undergraduate curriculum, and has now been taken up by other medical schools in the UK. This Internet module is designed 'for those with no prior knowledge about human rights as they impact on the practice of medicine'. It deals with issues that include medical involvement in torture, the diagnosis and rehabilitation of torture victims, doctors' involvement in the death penalty, human rights and public health, women's rights and rape in war, as well as mechanisms of redress for human rights abuses in member states of the European Community and those seeking asylum. The module has been used in Russia, India and Israel to teach human rights to lawyers and scientists, as well as to medical students. It has also been incorporated by the Centre for Enquiry into Health and Allied Themes (CEHAT) into a one-year diploma in the Civics and Politics Department of Bombay University, and into an intercalated BSc in International Health at the University College London.

Another initiative that differs from other available options is one that cuts across the boundaries of academe and makes no distinction between undergraduate and postgraduate status, the younger or older participant, but seeks rather to educate those working, or contemplating work, in the field of humanitarian crisis relief. The International Diploma in Humanitarian Assistance, which is conferred by the Center for International Health and Co-operation at Fordham University, the Royal College of Surgeons in Ireland and the University of Geneva, has been conferred on more than 400 graduates from over eighty nations. This one-month intensive residential course has a distinguished faculty that comprehensively covers the ethical and human rights aspects of humanitarian assistance including, among many topics, the historical background to humanitarian assistance, coping with humanitarian crises and protecting human rights, international law and human rights, planning and management of humanitarian relief in strife-torn communities, preventive diplomacy, law and ethics, environmental health, torture, landmines, trauma, sexual violence and rape, the military aspects to humanitarian crisis, the role of the media and the psychological and personal health of international relief workers.

If the growing imperative for teaching human rights to medical students is to be achieved, rhetoric and the passing of international resolutions will not solve the problem. The biggest difficulty for the deans of medical schools will not be any lack of acknowledgment of the importance of human rights for the doctors gradu-ating from their medical schools, or indeed of willingness to introduce the subject, but rather the impossibility of implementing a meaningful and well-structured course without having suitable teachers. In this regard medical schools would do well to take heed of what has been achieved in the Open University with distance learning, and the international experts in human rights would do well to pool their expertise in producing electronic learning modules in medical ethics and human rights for incorporation into the undergraduate curricula of medical schools across the world. In this regard, it is of relevance to note that European Biomed funding was obtained in 1996 to produce distance-learning workbooks on core themes in medical ethics for use across Europe. This project, known as the European Biomedical Ethics Practitioner Education (EBEPE) project was co-ordinated by the Imperial College School of Medicine in London in partnership with the Instituut voor Gezondheidsethiek in Maastricht, the Istituto Psicoanalitico per le Ricerche Sociali in Rome, the Zentrum für Ethik in der Medizin in Freiburg and the Department of Philosophy at the University of Turku in Finland. The training pack was published in 1999 with the objective of encouraging health professionals to assess differing approaches to resolving dilemmas, by illustrating how the same ethical challenges are handled in different European countries.

In concluding it would not be unreasonable to ask if there is any evidence that the teaching of human rights to medical students makes them better doctors. Intuitively my response would be affirmative but we live in a world where evidence is demanded for all statements, and to be fair the incorporation of human rights in the medical school curricula, as I have stressed, is not one to be undertaken lightly. A few international surveys have indeed shown that the teaching of human rights to medical students does increase awareness by allowing doctors to detach themselves from the prejudicial influences of their social background, but where doctors are faced with human rights abuse, education alone will not solve their dilemmas and the need for collegiate support then becomes necessary. More evidence on the value of teaching human rights is clearly needed but in fairness may be difficult to obtain, at least until the teaching of the subject is standardized to be made to comply with internationally accepted minimum standards.

If medicine with its long-established tradition of caring has been slow in acknowledging human rights, I hope I have not so much excused the profession for its shortcomings in this regard, but rather enunciated the real difficulties it faces in achieving what it recognizes as an urgent imperative. The Symposium 'Traditions, Values and Humanitarian Action' has served as a timely stimulus to assess the place of humanitarian action within the tradition of medicine, not merely as an audit of the current state of affairs within the undergraduate curriculum, but as the impetus to develop structures for the future implementation of human rights in the training of doctors. The teaching of human rights will not, of course, abolish the worldwide abuse of human rights, but it is an essential component in the fight to make the world a better place for all to live.

The Weight of Concern

IN 2011 Professor Damian McCormack published a letter in *The Irish Times* in which he deplored the fate of doctors who had been imprisoned in Bahrain when the wave of prodemocracy protest and revolution – the Arab Spring – engulfed that little island in February 2011.[39] I harboured affection for the island of Dilmun, which I had visited many years earlier when I had been a member of the academic staff of RCSI.[40] Now that College (and the Royal College of Physicians of Ireland) was prepared to stand by without protest while forty-seven doctors in Bahrain were imprisoned without trial and subjected to torture. All this might have little interest for Ireland were it not for the fact that some of the imprisoned doctors had been trained in Dublin and were fellows of RCSI, and that RCSI had invested heavily in building and staffing a medical university in Bahrain, known as RCSI-Bahrain. This university had been founded in 2004 on the authority of the government of the Kingdom of Bahrain, and the university campus was officially opened on 3 February 2009 by His Highness the prime minister of the Kingdom of Bahrain, Sh. Khalifa Bin Salman Al Khalifa and the then president of Ireland, Mary McAleese.

The largely peaceful protests in February 2011 demanded (in addition to an end to corruption and respect for human rights) not the overthrow of the monarchy but rather the establishment of a 'genuine' constitutional monarchy.[41] Indeed, in contrast to so many other Arab states, the essential structures for such a democratic process were in place. In 2002 King Hamad bin Isa Al Khalifa, who had succeeded his father as absolute ruler in 1999, introduced a system that included the establishment of a bicameral parliament with upper and lower houses. The problem with this democratic model is that it is not operated democratically. The upper house of forty seats is directly appointed by the king, and the lower house (also forty seats) is filled by an electoral constituency gerrymandering system that ensures that the Shia majority can never win more than twenty of the forty seats in spite of being 70 per cent of the population; the government is also directly appointed by the king.

Moreover, the prime minister Prince Khalifa bin Salman Al Khalifa, the king's uncle, has been in office for forty-seven years, and is the longest serving unelected head of government in the world. In March 2011 the king declared a state of emergency and invoked the Gulf Co-operation Council security agreements, which led to troops from Saudi Arabia and other gulf states being sent into the country, where they bulldozed public rallying points, including the Pearl Square, which has become a symbol of the protest movement. On 3 May the Military Public Prosecution charged twenty-four doctors and twenty-three nurses and paramedics with various offences based on 'investigation results' and 'confessions by some of the defendants'. It was alleged that in the course of obtaining these confessions, which were video-taped, serious violations in contravention of Bahraini and international human rights standards occurred, which included arbitrary arrest and detention, torture, abduction, beating, verbal abuse, being held incommunicado in solitary confinement during which time they were reportedly tortured and ill treated, apparently to force them to confess to the charges levelled against them.

Members of the medical profession in Ireland were particularly disturbed by the failure of both RCSI and the Royal College of Physicians of Ireland (RCPI) to speak out against the repression of doctors. I resigned my fellowship of RCPI in protest against the failure of the president of RCPI, who had been present at the joint conferring of degrees in RCSI Bahrain, to denounce the imprisonment without trial and alleged torture of medical personnel.

Madam, I write as a graduate and former member of the academic staff of the Royal College of Surgeons in Ireland (RCSI) and as a Fellow of the Royal College of Physicians of Ireland (RCPI) and as one who has written several books and many articles upholding the proud traditions of these institutions, to express my sadness and sense of shame, indeed betrayal, at seeing the presidents of both these institutions on a dais above the 1784 motto of RCSI *Consilio Manuque* (Scholarship and Dexterity) and beneath the banner 'Under the patronage of His Royal Highness Prince Khalifa bin Salman Al

Khalifa, the Prime Minister' at the graduation ceremony of the Royal College of Surgeons in Ireland-Medical University of Bahrain (RCSI Bahrain) on June 13th, 2011.

This action betrays the reality that doctors, some of who are graduates of RCSI, and nurses are in prison where some have been tortured and all of who face serious sentences, while the Royal Colleges excuse themselves from lending support by claiming to be non-political organizations.

Such an attitude is anathema to those of us who believe that the traditions of medicine must be upheld however unpleasant the consequence, which in this case is simply a large investment by RCSI in the medical school in Bahrain.

I can do little other than protest to the council and fellows of RCSI but I can express my concern in a more direct way to RCPI by resigning as a fellow. I have today written to the president Dr John Donohoe, tendering my resignation in protest against the failure of either Royal College to support colleagues who have been prevented from performing the fundamental duty that doctors are trained for, namely treating the sick and wounded. Eoin O'Brien.[42]

Front Line Defenders organized a delegation of concerned individuals from Ireland to visit Bahrain and I was invited as one of the representatives. Before going to Bahrain I asked the presidents of RCSI and RCPI to meet me. The latter did not respond to my letter but the president (Ms Eilis McGovern) and the vice-president (Mr Paddy Broe) of RCSI agreed to meet me and to discuss Bahrain. During this meeting I pleaded with the College to acknowledge that its stance was at variance with much national and international opinion. The plight of the imprisoned doctors had been condemned by doctors in Ireland and by international humanitarian groups. However, the College was adamant that its approach of so-called 'quiet diplomacy' as distinct from the approach advocated by me of outright condemnation of the way these doctors and nurses had been treated, was the correct course. The vice-president informed me that the imprisoned doctors, who happened to be fellows of RCSI, had obtained their fellowships many years earlier and besides they were 'not in good standing', a term with which I was unfamiliar, but which I was informed meant that they had not paid an annual fee so as to remain in the College network. The president likened the Fellowship to an accountancy examination from which she reasoned that the College had no more responsibility or obligations for its fellows than other institutions that conferred postgraduate recognition of achievement.

I expressed astonishment at this attitude, believing that if doctors trained in Dublin for their fellowship and paid the substantial fees for sitting the examination, it conferred exactly what the name suggests – the joining of a fellowship that could be expected to stand up for the principles of being able to practice surgery according to certain standards without fear or hindrance. The vice-president added that some of the arrested doctors were guilty of using medicine for political reasons, which I saw as a dangerous denigration of the principle of 'innocent until proven guilty'. The president explained to me the College's delicate relationship with the Bahraini authorities and the Arabic sense of conviction and that if the College denounced the treatment of doctors the College would be expelled from Bahrain. I begged to disagree pointing out that the College could, on the one hand, uphold the inalienable right of doctors to practice without fear or intimidation while also fulfilling the valuable role of providing medical education in the Middle East.

Both the president and vice-president suggested that if I had, as I had stated in my writings on the subject, a genuine affection for the College I would be supportive of the College's stance because the publicity surrounding this issue was doing irreparable damage to the College. I reasserted that my affection for the College was indeed genuine, both my parents and I being graduates, and that I had worked very hard over the years not only to elevate the College by writing its history but also by contributing to its scientific advancement, and that my meeting with them attested to a genuine desire to find an approach that would allow the College to secure its fiscal interests in Bahrain while also upholding the principles of medical practice. However, I emphasized that my affection could not extend to upholding a policy that was so convinced of its own self-righteousness as to be unable to consider alternative approaches.[43]

My account of the Front Line visit to Bahrain was published in *Irish Examiner*[44] and *The Lancet*.[45] Since this visit RCSI, while continuing to justify its stance, has had to retract and apologize for its actions. At least one imprisoned lecturer was suspended from her duties in RCSI-Bahrain. Then RCSI-Bahrain, which is staffed by several eminent academics and clinicians from Ireland, called in students identified in the protests to sign affidavits that they would not participate in political demonstrations and would swear an oath of loyalty to the king. How these students were identified, and by whom, has not been revealed but one must conclude that information passed between RCSI-Bahrain and the government.

The Chief Executive Officer of RCSI, Professor Cathal Kelly, has admitted that serious untoward events happened, among which was the demand from senior staff at the RCSI Bahrain that three medical students attending its college swear an oath of loyalty to the Bahraini Royal Family and sign, moreover, a declaration that they would not participate in political protests. RCSI has offered a series of belated platitudes: 'We have not lived up to the high standards that we set ourselves in these matters ... actions were unacceptable and should never have happened ... actions might appear insensitive and open to misinterpretation ...

questions were wholly inappropriate and inconsistent with our ethos.' The new president of RCSI-Bahrain 'unreservedly apologized' to the students who were forced to swear allegiance to the king by staff of RCSI-Bahrain and he has returned to the students the signed and witnessed documents.[46]

In fairness to RCSI, it has a significant financial interest in Bahrain and it has taken a stance, albeit one that it has had to modify in the light of developments and revelations, but the silence of its sister college RCPI is truly inexcusable. The only statement that I am aware of was made by the outgoing president, Dr John Donohoe, who stated that RCPI was aware (*mirabile dictu*) 'that many of our Fellows have been particularly shocked by the events unfolding in Bahrain' and then he belatedly reiterated what has been said so ably by concerned individuals and international bodies that 'it was essential that the judicial process underway in relation to these medical professionals had to be demonstrably and unequivocally fair and just, and be seen to arrive at the truth of what really happened'.[47] This fatuous statement is all the more remarkable when it has been clearly shown by the Bahrain Independent Commission of Inquiry (BICI), that the Public Security Forces violated human rights by forcibly entering and ransacking houses without arrest warrants, and subjecting detainees to blindfolding, enforced standing for prolonged periods, electrocution, sleep-deprivation, and threats of rape with the purpose of obtaining incriminating statements or confessions.

Taken with forensic medical evidence the BICI adjudged that torture was common and that such practices were a flagrant disregard both of Bahrain and international human rights law. However daunting these criticisms may be for the security forces' use of internecine practices, a more worrying aspect for the many doctors and others in Bahrain who still stand accused and who are still being tried, is the serious criticism of the Bahrain judicial system by the BICI, which must call into question the validity of sentences previously passed. The commission viewed the 'lack of accountability' of the judicial and prosecutorial personnel in the National Safety Court as 'a subject of great concern', compounded by the acceptance of forced confessions in criminal proceedings in both special courts and ordinary criminal courts. The commissioners went on to recommend that sentences should be dropped, or at least reviewed, for those charged with offences involving political expression, or victims of torture, ill-treatment or prolonged incommunicado detention, and that victims of human rights abuse should be compensated, and that dismissed employees should be reinstated and compensated. This recommendation has not been enacted and the farcical trials of doctors continue in Bahrain.[48]

The Island of Dilmun, 1989

In Dilmun the raven utters no cry,
the wild hen utters not the cry of the wild hen,
the lion kills not,
the wolf snatches not the lamb,
unknown is the kid-devouring wild dog,
unknown is the grain-devouring boar.

Enki and Ninhursag
(Sumerian poem *c.*4000 BC)

ANYONE WHO HAS READ Geoffrey Bibby's *Looking for Dilmun: The Search for a Lost Civilization* must yearn to visit the island of Dilmun, 'the place where the sun rises'. For me it was not only the Arab culture that beckoned, but there was also one more ancient culture, one dating from the early Bronze Age of the third millennium BC, which had chosen the island of Bahrain as a paradise, a land of beauty for immortals, an island that was to become the largest prehistoric cemetery in the world, sealing in stone and sand the mortal evidence of a bygone age in 170,000 burial mounds. Here, I believed, was to be found another Tír na nÓg, a land of peace and beauty, of legend and myth, an island of potsherds, passage graves, raths and tumuli, the chastening evidence that greatness existed before our time, that man's mind has always soared on a dream and that the heights attained are dependent only on how high above the clouds the dreamer's fantasy reaches. Bahrain was all of this and much more.

The College of Surgeons, in choosing Bahrain for the historic occasion of its first overseas meeting, chose wisely. Bahrain, though an Arab country espousing the Islamic religion, has acquired by virtue of its unique role as host over may centuries to traders and visitors from all parts of the world, a sense of hospitality that accepts the customs and traditions that are foreign to its own, while at the same time retaining the Arabian tradition that imparts to the island its own unique character. This balance is difficult to attain and other Islamic states have found it necessary to take measures, in varying degrees, to protect their culture. It would be well for visitors to the Middle East to recognize that there are some extremely undesirable attributes to the ethos they bring with them, not least of which is the discourtesy of propounding on Islamic religious customs without having taken the trouble to try to understand their complex origins and development, and to which the greatest threat must be the influence of the awesome banality of American television.

However, surely the greatest disservice by western civilizations must have been the attempted exploitation of Arab hospitality and relatively new-found wealth without any thought for the consequences of such avarice on the development of this strategic part of the world. It would be disingenuous in this regard to fail to observe that the medical profession has not always behaved with the decorum commensurate with its perceived role as one that espouses humanitarian ideals and from which a certain spirit of altruism might not be inappropriate. The past tense is, hopefully, apt, as there is ample evidence to indicate that the Arabian countries have come to terms with the problems that beset all bounty.

It may be well to note that Arab memory is not short. Friends are fondly cherished, the charlatan is soon recognized and, in time, expropriated. It would be the wish of the College to rank among the former, for its influence has been considerable and constructive. In medical education, the College and Ireland have played a substantial role in Kuwait, Iraq, Bahrain, Qatar, Saudi Arabia, the United Arab Emirates, Oman and Sudan, but it is through the undergraduate and post-graduate alumni of the medical school that the College will exert a lasting and beneficial impact on the health of these and neighbouring countries. The Minister for Health, Mr Jawad Salem Al-Arayed, in acknowledging the influence of over forty Irish trained doctors and nurses in Bahrain, paid tribute to the College for holding a conference that exemplified one of the College's major attributes, namely a forum whereby countries of diverse cultures were brought together to exchange knowledge in the education of doctors for the treatment of mankind, and in the achievement of which race, nationality, religion and status should be of no concern. If all educational endeavours embraced these values, the essence of Islam 'peace be with you' would be acknowledged.

The meeting in Bahrain served as an opportunity for surgeons from the Gulf States to exchange ideas relating to the development of surgery in their countries with their Irish colleagues, and this exchange of views is of sufficient interest to merit publication, if for no other reason than to illustrate for us the enormous health-care problems that must be dealt with in the Middle East.

The social highlights of the meeting are outlined elsewhere in this issue. I nurture three memories that shall endure. First, I had the good fortune to be intro-duced casually in the Souk to the Superintendent of Archaeology for the State of Bahrain, Abdulaziz Ali Sowaileh, who on hearing of my interest in the Dilmun dynasty took a small group of us around the more recent excavations. We were priv-ileged to experience the remarkable sensation that accompanies the gentle dusting away of the last layer of sand to reveal a piece of pottery or an exquisite ring with an agate set in silver dating from 3000 years. Such is the stuff of archaeology and how enlightening it was to see a policy of excavation that obliged the bulldozers of commerce to stand by while the archaeologists, under the experienced and watchful eye of Abdulaziz, painstakingly excavated and carefully archived their historic treasures for later display in a museum presently being built. Would that our philistinic city fathers, who permitted the desecration of Wood Quay, might take note of the policies being enacted on another small island with a rich historic legacy.

My second lasting memory is of the hospitality shown to me by Essa Amin in his home and that of his mother where I glimpsed, hopefully not for the last time, the magic of a culture quite foreign to my own. Such is the essence of travel and herein lies the importance of meetings such as this first overseas meeting of the College in that the visitor is afforded the opportunity to give but more can be received than is ever given in that the traveller's perception of the unfamiliar, of the hitherto unknown, is enriched by a deeper understanding and a broadening of outlook.

I left Bahrain pondering the future of the land of Dilmun with a degree of pessimism, not because of anything obviously perceptible in the island now, but because of the vulnerable honesty of a local taxi driver, who in restoring to me my sunglasses, which I had assumed lost when I left them in his car the day before, assured me that nothing was ever stolen in Bahrain. To emphasize the point, he told me how a road-sweeper some months earlier had found, in the course of his labours, a packet containing some thousands of dollars by the kerbside of a bank where a wealthy foreigner had dropped it, and he had taken this precious trove representing more than he could hope to amass in two lifetimes to the bank. I, too, remembered a day when doors needed not locks and the old could live on their holdings in the countryside without fear of molestation. If one island culture had lost all this and much more in what might be euphemistically termed its emancipation, why not another? And yet there is something about the resilience of the Arab personality that leads me to think, to hope, that this will be otherwise. The world will be the poorer if it is not so.

Bahrain – Continuing Imprisonment of Doctors, 2011

THE WAVE of pro-democracy protest and revolution in many Arab states – the Arab Spring – reached Bahrain in February 2011. The protest was soon ruthlessly suppressed with the help of forces from Saudi Arabia. Bahrain's main public hospital, the Salmaniya Medical Complex, was subsequently occupied by the military. Several independent observers recorded the brutality of the clampdown, reports of imprisonment, torture, extraction of confessions, and the military trials. More than seventy medical professionals, including forty-seven doctors, were arrested and more than 150 medical workers have been suspended or dismissed from their jobs.

Ireland's close medical relation with Bahrain, which extends back many years, took on a new dimension when the Royal College of Surgeons in Ireland (RCSI) invested almost €100 million to develop the RCSI–Medical University of Bahrain. In June 2011, when RCSI and the Royal College of Physicians of Ireland conferred joint degrees in Bahrain, the failure of either College's president to visit the families of the imprisoned doctors, some of whom had trained in Dublin and were fellows of RCSI, drew strong protest from the medical profession in Ireland. Subsequently the international human rights organization Front Line Defenders organized a delegation from Ireland to visit Bahrain to offer support to these medical personnel. The delegation comprised two doctors, Damian McCormack and myself; three politicians, Averil Power, Senator of the Irish Parliament, David Andrews, former Minister for Foreign Affairs, and Marian Harkin, Member of the European Parliament; two members of Front Line Defenders, Andrew Anderson and Khalid Ibrahim; and a photojournalist, Conor McCabe.

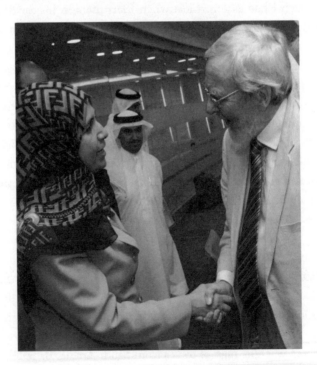

Fatima Al Balushi, Bahrain's Minister of Human Rights and acting Minister of Health, with the author in Bahrain, 2011.

During a two-day visit we met the administration of the Salmaniya Medical Complex, representatives of the Ministry of Foreign Affairs, and Fatima Al Balushi, Minister of Human Rights and Social Development and acting Minister of Health. In our preamble to these meetings we indicated that although many similarities existed between Ireland and Bahrain, freedom of speech was a cornerstone of Ireland's democracy, and accused persons were innocent until proven guilty. Al Balushi expressed her pride in the human rights achievements in Bahrain, especially in furthering the rights of women and religious freedom. Al Balushi said that the Arab Spring had brought the country to the verge of civil war. She claimed that several doctors had failed to care for the wounded and must therefore face trial. Asked if the allegations of kidnapping, detention, and torture were true, she answered that if such was found to be the case, the perpetrators would be duly prosecuted. She acknowledged that mistakes had been made but said that these had been redressed by the king with the appointment of an independent commission to investigate violations of human rights, the transfer of trials from military to civilian courts, and the release of medical detainees who were not a threat to national security. Al Balushi agreed to approach the king with a request on our behalf for the release of detained doctors (a request that has not been granted to date and many imprisoned doctors are now reported to be on hunger strike); she asked in return that I give Bahrain fair coverage in *The Lancet*, which she regarded as being unfairly biased against Bahrain.

Our delegation went to secret locations to meet members of the families of imprisoned doctors and doctors who had been released pending trial, and to meet ambulance drivers who said they had been taken from their ambulances, imprisoned, and tortured. Some of those who said they had been imprisoned were clearly suffering from anxiety, emotional instability, and depression. The loyalty and affection expressed by doctors suspended from the Salmaniya Medical Complex, where so many of them had served for many years, contrasted strongly with their feeling of betrayal by RCSI–Bahrain. We also met Nabeel Rajab, president of the Bahrain Centre for Human Rights, and Abdulla Al Derazi, general secretary of the Bahrain Human Rights Society, who have each carefully documented instances of torture for submission to the relevant international human rights bodies.

At the end of our visit we were in no doubt that doctors and medical personnel had been subjected to human rights abuses, including kidnapping, detention without trial in solitary confinement, and the extraction of confessions under torture. We left Bahrain moved by their gratitude for our support and embarrassed that we were offering so little in the face of the enormity of their suffering and courage. The medical community worldwide needs to take notice and speak out for colleagues who are being denied basic human rights, and who are being subjected to indignities that the medical profession should not tolerate.

Doctors in Bahrain Merit More than Platitudes, 2011

MUCH HAS HAPPENED in the small island of Bahrain since it was engulfed in the Arab Spring in February. Unlike other conflicts in other Arab states, the Bahrain protest did not demand the downfall of the ruling regime but sought the establishment of a democratic constitutional monarchy and recognition of human rights.

The protest was brutally suppressed when the king sought the assistance of Saudi-led forces in March. More than thirty-five people were killed and forty-seven doctors were among at least 1000 citizens imprisoned without trial, tortured, charged in military courts and condemned to preposterous sentences.

In July a delegation from Ireland visited Bahrain and reported unequivocally that the accused doctors had endured serious abuses of human rights that included torture, and called for the relevant authorities in Ireland to support them. At the time King Hamad bin Isa Al Khalifa also established an independent commission of inquiry to investigate the events in Bahrain during and after the Arab Spring protests and to make recommendations. The 500-page report, presented to the king last week, was based on evidence from over 8000 complaints and interviews with over 5000 individuals.

The report begins by emphasizing that Bahrain is party to a number of international human rights treaties, which obliges the kingdom to adhere to certain standards and that when human rights violations occur the perpetrators must be held accountable.

On the charges against the doctors the commissioners are ambiguous in their assessment of events at the Salmaniya Medical Complex. They were clearly faced with the dilemma of having to reconcile the possibility that some doctors were involved in political activities with the fact that the security forces executed unlawful arrests on the hospital premises, attacked and mistreated medical personnel, and confined injured patients in a special ward.

The commissioners had no hesitation in accusing the Public Security Forces of violating human rights by forcibly entering and sometimes ransacking houses without arrest warrants, and terrifying the occupants. There is an abundance of documented evidence that detainees were subjected, among many abuses, to blindfolding, enforced standing for prolonged periods, electrocution, sleep deprivation, and threats of rape with the purpose of obtaining incriminating statements or confessions.

Taken with forensic medical evidence the commission adjudged that torture was common and that such practices were a flagrant disregard both of Bahrain and international human rights law. Perhaps one of the most important aspects of the report is the serious criticism of the Bahrain judicial system, which must call into question the validity of sentences passed. The commission viewed the 'lack of accountability' of the judicial and prosecutorial personnel in the National Safety Court as 'a subject of great concern', compounded by the acceptance of forced confessions in criminal proceedings in both special courts and ordinary criminal courts.

The commission recommendations were far-reaching and must leave many Bahrainis fearing the retributive consequences that must ensue if they are enacted. The government is to establish a national independent and impartial mechanism to determine the accountability of those in government who have committed unlawful or negligent acts resulting in the deaths, torture and mistreatment of civilians with a view to bringing legal and disciplinary action against such individuals, including those in the chain of command, military and civilian, who are found to be responsible under international standards of superior responsibility.

The commissioners recommend that death sentences for murder be commuted, that charges should be dropped, or at least reviewed, for victims of torture, ill-treatment or prolonged incommunicado detention; that victims of human rights abuse be compensated, and that dismissed employees be reinstated and compensated. Finally, the commissioners warn that 'the state should never again resort to detention without prompt access to lawyers' and access to the outside world.

The commissioners must be commended for their thoroughness.

However, it is disappointing that the report does not name and blame the person or persons in charge of, for example, the Public Security Forces, which have been implicated in many of the atrocities.

It is to be hoped that the government will not resort to making minor police officers scapegoats but rather identify the people in high places – perhaps even in the royal family – who condoned or ordered the brutal behaviour of those under their command.

Given the ineptitude of the legal system it is difficult to see how the charges and sentences that have been passed can be legally upheld.

Concerned doctors in Ireland have voiced their criticism of the Royal College of Surgeons in Ireland (RCSI) and the Royal College of Physicians for failing to support colleagues in Bahrain. The report vindicates those from Ireland who supported the accused doctors and their families. By the same token the report emphasizes the failure of the colleges to join with international humanitarian groups, such as Front Line Defenders, Médecins Sans Frontières, Human Rights Watch and Physicians for Human Rights in condemning the Bahraini authorities.

As a result the colleges have been criticized by *The Lancet* and the *British Medical Journal,* two of the world's most widely read medical journals, with the latter accusing RCSI-Bahrain of complicity with the regime.

Under such pressure RCSI acknowledges that its 'actions were unacceptable and should never have happened'. But platitudinous statements are not good enough; the Royal Colleges have damaged Ireland's hard-earned reputation in medicine internationally and it is to be hoped that when doctors and nurses are threatened in areas of future unrest and political upheaval, these institutions will staunchly support the principle of medical neutrality.

References

PART ONE

See www.eoinobrien.org for further references

1. The Beckett Country Exhibition has been displayed at thirty venues worldwide, which include the MacRobert Art Gallery, University of Stirling, Scotland; the Atrium, Trinity College, Dublin; the Olivier Gallery, National Theatre, London; Théâtre du Rond-Point, Paris; Kenny's Art Gallery, Galway; the Royal Hospital, Kilmainham; the Belltable, Limerick; the Town Hall, Castlebar; the Town Hall, Dundalk; the Ardhowen Theatre, Enniskillen; the Ulster Museum, Belfast; Clifden Arts Festival, Galway; the Irish College, Louvain; Aachen University, Bonn; Biblioteca Nacional, Madrid; New York Public Library; University of New Orleans; Statten Gallery, Emory University, Atlanta; Sulzer Regional Library, Chicago; Beaumont Hospital, Dublin; The Gate Theatre, Dublin; Maison de la Poésie, Théâtre Molière, Paris; Bibliothèque Municipale de Strasbourg; Maison de la Fontaine, Brest; Université de Caen; the Dublin Writer's Museum; Dundalk Institute of Technology; County Hall, Dún Laoghaire; the University of Leuven; and is now on permanent loan to the James Joyce Library at University College Dublin.

2. E. O'Brien, 'The Weight of Compassion' was first published in French as 'Samuel Beckett et le Poids de la Compassion' in *Critique* 66 (1990) pp. 641–53, as translated by Edith Fournier, whose advice in preparing this text for publication I acknowledge with gratitude; and in English as 'Samuel Beckett and the Weight of Compassion', *The Recorder* 10 (1997), pp. 154–65.

3. E. O'Brien, 'The Beckett Country: Samuel Beckett's Ireland' was first published as the Introduction to E. O'Brien, *The Beckett Country: Samuel Beckett's Ireland* (Black Cat Press in association with Faber and Faber, London and New York, 1986), pp. xix–xxvi. The text has been modified for this publication.

4. E. O'Brien, 'Zone of Stones', the sixteenth Arnold K. Henry Lecture in the Royal College of Surgeons in Ireland on 9 October 1996; an illustrated lecture based on E. O'Brien, *The Beckett Country*. First published in the *Journal of the Irish Colleges of Physicians and Surgeons* 16 (1987), pp. 69–77. The audio-visual production *Zone of Stones: Samuel Beckett's Dublin* was compiled and narrated by Eoin O'Brien, with photography by David Davison and sound by Patrick Duffner. Permission to reprint

excerpts and quotations was kindly granted by Samuel Beckett, John Calder, Faber and Faber and the Black Cat Press.

5. E. O'Brien, 'Humanity in Ruins' was first published in the *Journal of the Irish Colleges of Physicians and Surgeons* 19 (1990), pp. 137–45. See also: E. O'Brien, *The Beckett Country*, pp. 314–42 and pp. 383–6. Since this essay was published, Phyllis Gaffney (daughter of James Gaffney), who is senior lecturer at the School of Languages and Literature at University College Dublin, has written *Healing Amid the Ruins: the Irish Hospital at Saint-Lô 1945–1946* (A&A Farmar, Dublin, 1999).

6. E. O'Brien, 'From the Waters of Zion to Liffeyside', *Journal of the Irish Colleges of Physicians and Surgeons* 10 (1981), pp. 107–19. The twelfth Leonard Abrahamson Memorial Lecture was delivered in the Royal College of Surgeons on 13 March 1980. My researches for this essay were greatly facilitated by a few people whose help it gives me pleasure to acknowledge. Niall Sheridan, whose love of Jewish humour and fascination for Jewish culture he was privileged to share with James Joyce in Paris. My friendship with the late Con Leventhal in Paris and Ivor Radnor in Birmingham gave me a deeper insight into the character of the Dublin Jew than books could ever do. Leonard's brother Dr Mervyn Abrahamson in London supplied me with much valuable material. In Dublin, Jack Lyons, Michael Solomons, Serge Philipson, Joe Briscoe and Colin Simon helped me in my researches.

7. E. O'Brien, 'The Writings of A.J. Leventhal' was first published as 'The Writings of A.J. Leventhal, a Bibliography' in E. O'Brien (ed.), *A.J. Leventhal, 1896–1979, Dublin Scholar, Wit and Man of Letters* (Leventhal Scholarship Committee, The Glendale Press, Dublin, 1984), pp. 19–31, and later as 'The Writings of A.J. Leventhal: a Bibliography', *The Recorder* 8 (1995), pp. 48–64. A bibliography of the Dramatic Commentary series by A.J. Leventhal in *The Dublin Magazine* between 1943 and 1958 can be found in these publications.

8. The essay on Nevill Johnson is based on D. Hall and E. O'Brien, *Nevill Johnson: Paint the Smell of Grass* (Ava Gallery, Northern Ireland, 2008).

9. N. Sheridan, 'Doctors and Literature', *British Medical Journal* 2 (1978), pp. 1779–80.

10. The essay on Denis Johnston is based on 'Nine Rivers from Jordan' in the Medicine and Books Reading for Pleasure series in *British Medical Journal* 2 (1978), pp. 1408–9.

11. The essay on Mícheál MacLiammóir is based on 'On the Saint Patrick', *British Medical Journal* 2 (1978), pp. 187–8.

12. E. O'Brien, 'Obituary of Petr Skrabanek', *British Medical Journal* 309 (1994), p. 184.

13. E. O'Brien, 'A Vindication of Petr Skrabanek', *Irish Medical Times* (31 July 1998), p. 25.

14. T. Sherwood, 'Ombudsman's Second Report, and Tobacco', *The Lancet* 352 (1998), p. 7–8.

15. R. Fox, 'Petr Skrabanek and *The Lancet*', *Journal of Clinical Epidemology*, 49 (1996), pp. 607–8.

16. The essay on Petr Skrabanek is based on E. O'Brien, '*The Cantos of Maldoror* by Comte de Lautréamont', *The Recorder* 10 (1997), pp. 57–65.

17. E. O'Brien, 'History of the Blood Pressure Unit at the Charitable Infirmary and

Beaumont Hospital 1978–2006', *Heartwise* (Winter 2006), pp. 12–18. Scientific papers from the Unit can be found on www.eoinobrien.org.

18. The essay on Anton Chekhov is based on 'The Little-Known Compassion of Dr Anton Chekhov', *The Lancet* 352 (1988), pp. 331–3, a review of J. Coope, *Doctor Chekhov: A Study in Literature and Medicine* (Cross Publishing, Isle of Wight, 1997).

19. The essay on Nikolai Korotkoff is based on M. Laher and E. O'Brien (eds.), 'In Search of Nikolai Korotkoff', *British Medical Journal*, 285 (1982), pp. 1796–8. This essay is based on the researches of Dr Harold Segall and especially of his illustrated monograph on Korotkoff. His generosity in providing much biographical detail, advice and illustrations for the essay is acknowledged, as is the assistance of Mr Frank Edwards, honorary secretary of the Ireland-USSR Society, who translated several papers from the Russian.

20. The essay on George Frideric Handel is based on an essay by E. O'Brien in the programme of the recital of *Messiah: An Oratorio* in aid of the Medical Research Fund of The Charitable Infirmary and the Mercer Hospital Development Fund in the National Concert Hall, Dublin in 1986 (Black Cat Press, Dublin, 1986).

21. The essay on Dominic Corrigan is based on 'The Dublin School and the Golden Age of Irish Medicine' in E. O'Brien, *Conscience and Conflict: A Biography of Sir Dominic Corrigan 1802–1880* (Glendale Press, Dublin, 1983), pp. 107–70, and E. O'Brien, *A Century of Service: The City of Dublin Skin and Cancer Hospital 1911–2012* (The Anniversary Press, Dublin, 2011).

22. The essay 'Some Irish Doctors in Literature' is based on E. O'Brien, 'Let Verse and Humour be Our Music' in E. O'Brien, L. Browne, K. O'Malley (eds.), *The House of Industry Hospitals, 1772–1987, The Richmond, Whitworth and Hardwicke (St Laurence's Hospital), A Closing Memoir* (Anniversary Press, Dublin, 1988), pp. 156–88.

23. The essay on Dom Peter Flood is based on the essay by E. O'Brien 'Lunch at Ealing Abbey; Dom Peter Flood', *Journal of the Irish Medical Association* 72 (1979), pp. 40–1.

PART TWO

1. E. O'Brien, 'Six Years Shalt Thou Labour', *World Medicine* (March 1979), pp. 26–7.

2. E. O'Brien, 'History, Diagnosis and *then* Examination', *Journal of the Irish Medical Association* 72 (1979), p. 499.

3. E. O'Brien, 'The Dangers of the Dublin Disease', inaugural meeting of the Biological Society of the Royal College of Surgeons in Ireland, 7 November 1981. First published as 'Towards Being a Scientific Doctor and the Dangers of the Dublin Disease', *Journal of the Irish Colleges of Physicians and Surgeons* 12 (1982), pp. 71–4.

4. E. O'Brien, A. Crookshank, G. Wolstenholme (eds.), *A Portrait of Irish Medicine; An Illustrated History of Medicine in Ireland* (Ward River Press and the Royal College of Surgeons in Ireland, Dublin, 1984).

5. 'The Royal College of Surgeons in Ireland, 1784–1984. The Architecture of an

Achievement from Charter to Bicentennial' in E. O'Brien, A. Crookshank, G. Wolstenholme (eds.), *A Portrait of Irish Medicine; An Illustrated History of Medicine in Ireland* (Ward River Press and RCSI, Dublin, 1984), pp. 287–95.

6. 'What is a Professor?' *Journal of the Irish Medical Association* 72 (1979), p. 358.

7. ' "In Dublin's Fair City", Walter Somerville: The Early Days', *British Heart Journal* 45 (1981), pp. 5–8.

8. E. O'Brien, *World Medicine* (1978), p. 31.

9. G. Sandler, *British Medical Journal* 2 (1979), p. 21.

10. F.A. Jones, *Richard Asher Talking Sense* (Pitman Medical, London, 1972), p. 179.

11. L. Witts, 'The Medical Professorial Unit', *British Medical Journal* 2 (1971), p. 319.

12. E. O'Brien, 'Two Colleges and a Medical School', *Journal of the Irish Colleges of Physicians and Surgeons* 8 (1979), p. 133.

13. E. O'Brien, 'The Bicentenary of the Royal College of Surgeons in Ireland, 1784–1984', *British Medical Journal* 287 (1983), pp. 1988–90.

14. E. O'Brien, 'The Royal College of Surgeons in Ireland: A Bicentennial Tribute', *Journal of the Irish Colleges of Physicians and Surgeons* 13 (1984), pp. 29–34.

15. J. O'Callaghan, unpublished letter to the Editor, *Journal of the Irish Colleges of Physicians and Surgeons*, 1984.

16. E. O'Brien, unpublished letter to the Editor, *Journal of the Irish Colleges of Physicians and Surgeons*, 1 October 1985.

17. E. O'Brien, 'Strike and the Medical Profession', *Irish Medical Journal* 80 (1987), pp. 247–8.

18. E. O'Brien, 'Closure of the *Irish Medical Journal*', *Irish Medical Journal* 80 (1987), pp. 335–6.

19. S. Lock, 'Editorial Freedom: a Modest Proposal to Dublin', *British Medical Journal* 296 (1988), pp. 733–4.

20. G.D. Lundberg, 'Editorial Freedom and Integrity', *Journal of the American Medical Association* 260 (1988), p. 2563.

21. J.F. Henahan, 'This St Patrick's Day Finds No Lack of Controversy at *Irish Medical Journal*', *Journal of the American Medical Association* 261 (1989), pp. 1543–9.

22. Anonymous, Editorial, *Journal of the Irish Free State Medical Union*, 1 (1937), p.1.

23. Anonymous, *The Lancet* 4 (1987), p. 1442.

24. E. O'Brien, R.D. Thornes, D. O'Brien, B. Hogan, 'Inhibition of Antiplasmin and Fibrinolytic Effect of Protease in Patients with Cancer', *The Lancet* 1 (1968), pp. 173–6.

25. Anonymous, 'Protease and Cancer', *The Lancet* 1 (1968), pp. 188–9.

26. 'Fourteenth Annual Clinical Meeting of the British Medical Association', *British Medical Journal* 2 (1971), p. 153.

27. 'Seventeenth Annual Clinical Meeting of the British Medical Association Held in Conjunction with the Medical Association of Jamaica', *British Medical Journal* 2 (1974), p. 313.

28. E. O'Brien, 'East Mediterranean Medical Congress', *Irish Medical Journal*, 65 (1972), pp. 234–5.

29. E. O'Brien, 'Or in the Heart or in the Head', *British Medical Journal* 4 (1976), p. 1158.

30. E. O'Brien, 'Will No-One Tell Me What She Sings?', *British Medical Journal* 4 (1976), p. 1091.

31. E. O'Brien, 'Coitus and Coronaries', *British Medical Journal* 14 (1976), p. 414.

32. E. O'Brien, 'Stephen Lock – Hibernian in Disguise', *The Brayer* in *British Medical Journal* (April 1991).

33. E. O'Brien, 'The Tragedy of the Medicine Man in the Underdeveloped World', *Journal of the Irish Colleges of Physicians and Surgeons* 18 (1989), pp. 22–3.

34. E. O'Brien, 'Walk in Peace: Banish Landmines from our Globe' *British Medical Journal* 315 (1997), pp. 1456–8.

35. E. O'Brien, 'The Diplomatic Implications of Emerging Diseases' in K.M. Cahill, *Preventive Diplomacy: Stopping Wars Before They Start* (BasicBooks, New York, 2000), pp. 244–68.

36. E. O'Brien, 'Human Rights and the Making of a Good Doctor' in K. Cahill, *Traditions, Values and Humanitarian Action* (International Humanitarian Series, Fordham University Press, New York, 2003), pp. 136–52.

37. Centre for International Humanitarian Cooperation, www.cihc.org.

38. G. Parati, S. Mendis, D. Abegunde, R. Asmar, S. Mieke, A. Murray, B. Shengelia, G. Steenvoorden, G. Van Montfrans, E. O'Brien, 'Recommendations for Blood Pressure Measuring Devices for Office/Clinic Use in Low Resource Setting', *Blood Pressure Monitoring* 10 (2005), pp. 3–10.

39. D. McCormack, 'Medics Held in Bahrain', *The Irish Times* (6 May 2011).

40. E. O'Brien, 'The Island of Dilmun', *Journal of the Irish Colleges of Physicians and Surgeons* 18 (1989), pp. 6–7.

41. S. Devi, 'Health Professionals Under Threat in Bahrain', *The Lancet* 377 (2011), pp. 1733–4.

42. E. O'Brien, 'Treatment of Medics in Bahrain', letter to *The Irish Times*, 6 June 2011.

43. Email from Eoin O'Brien to Ms Eilis McGovern, 7 October 2011.

44. E. O'Brien, 'Hippocratic Oath', *Irish Examiner* (2 August 2011), p. 13.

45. E. O'Brien, 'Bahrain: Continuing Imprisonment of Doctors', *The Lancet* 378 (2011), pp. 1203–4.

46. E. O'Brien, 'Doctors in Bahrain Merit More Than Platitudes', *The Irish Times* (29 November 2011), and 'Report Confirms Torture of Doctors', *Irish Medical Times* (9 December 2011).

47. Statement from outgoing Royal College of Physicians of Ireland President Dr John Donohoe on Bahrain to the Annual Stated Meeting of the Royal College of Physicians of Ireland, held 20 October 2011.

48. E. O'Brien, 'A Simple Question for Bahrain: Will the King of Bahrain Implement the Recommendations of the BICI?', *Irish Medical Times* (30 March 2012).

Index